The holistic
management
of horses

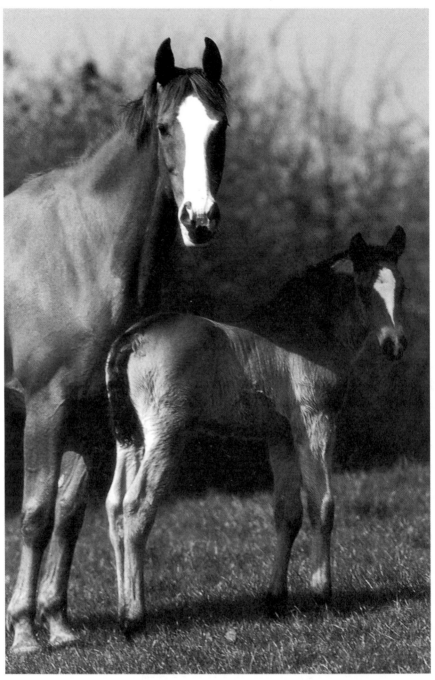

The domesticated horse relies entirely on mankind to provide for all its needs. Its health and welfare depend on proper husbandry.

The holistic management of horses

Keith Allison

Veterinary adviser
Christopher Day MRCVS

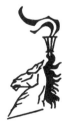

J. A. Allen
London

British Library Cataloguing in Publication Data
A catalogue record for this book is available from the British Library.

ISBN 0.85131.623.9

Published in Great Britain in 1996 by

J. A. Allen & Company Limited
1 Lower Grosvenor Place, London SW1W 0EL

Editor Elizabeth O'Beirne-Ranelagh
Designer Nancy Lawrence

Typeset in Hong Kong by Setrite Typesetters Ltd.
Printed in Hong Kong by Dah Hua Printing Press Co. Ltd.

To A.

When Allah willed to create the horse, he said to the south wind, 'condense theyself; I will that a creature shall proceed from thee'.

Contents

Acknowledgements

Illustrations on pp. 18 (bottom), 19, 23, 26, 40, 41, 42, 43, 44, 45, 47, 56, 57, 104, 107−11, 136, 139, 143, 145, 159, 160, 169, 171 and 173 from Prof. J. Wortley-Axe, *The Horse: its treatment in health and disease*, 9 vols. (London 1905−6).

Illustrations on pp. 38, 84, 89, 140, 146, 147, 148, 164, and 166 by Maggie Raynor.

Photographs on pp. ii. 2, 7, 30, 32, 38, 39, 48, 49, 54, 70, 75, 94, 133, 140, 141, 152, 155, 166, 168 and 175 copyright Bob Langrish.

Photographs on pp. 20, 32 and 86 kindly supplied by Mrs E. K. Winter.

Photograph on p. 113 kindly supplied by the Sir William Dunn School of Pathology, Oxford.

Photograph on p. 117 kindly supplied by Pennsylvania State University, USA.

Photograph on p. 138 kindly supplied by Mr E. Byrne.

1

The principles of holism

'Holism is not only creative, but self creative.'
Jan Christian Smuts (1870–1950)

Holism is based on the fundamental principle of nature, which is the creation and maintenance of wholes, or complete biological systems. Disharmony of any part of that system, no matter how small, has the potential to disrupt the integrity of the whole.

While this concept has been appreciated in many cultures through the ages, it was Jan Christian Smuts (1870–1950) who enabled it to be understood in modern scientific terms. He coined the term 'holism', and now years after his death the word is being used in many areas outside the natural sciences.

The theory of holism can be demonstrated in all matter, operating at all levels, from the atom and the cell to the most complicated biological systems. An example of the principle of holism can be seen in the immensely complex organisation and behaviour of individual biological cells, functioning for the good of the whole being.

The general use of the word 'holistic' describes a system of management which follows these overall principles. Therefore we may describe any practice concerned with equine husbandry as being 'holistic' if it is designed to take account of the maintenance of the whole.

The same general principles may be used to define holistic practices in medical and non-medical therapies; however, when we come to apply the word to feeding stuffs and supplements, it has a precise meaning (see p. 68).

One of the main reasons for the recent interest in holistic management of horses is that we are appreciating the benefits of

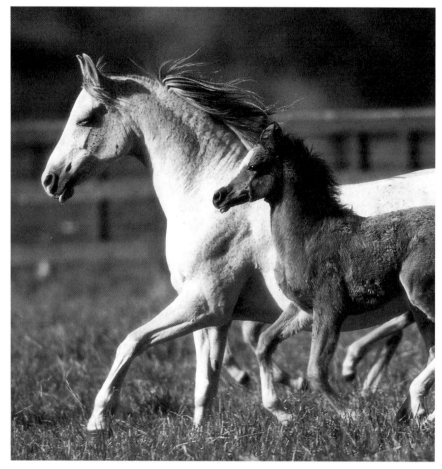

The beauty, grace and speed of the Arab horse has been prized for centuries. An investigation into equine pedigrees shows how important it has been in the development of many breeds of horses.

holism in our own lives. With our evolving attitude towards the health and welfare of the animals in our care we naturally wish to provide them with the same benefits.

An area in which there is much interest today is that of holistic nutrition and medicine. In the twentieth century we have tended to compartmentalise the two subjects, as we do many other disciplines. The holistic approach here is particularly effective, and easily understood, because of the close relationship between the two disciplines. There is no real difference between nutrition and medicine: anything taken by mouth has, or can have, an influence on the body. This is not a new revelation. It was discussed by Hippocrates (*c.* 460−377 BC), who is regarded by the modern world as 'the Father of Medicine'.

Today, where the more technical aspects of nutrition and medicine are involved, what should be a simple matter can be confusing. Modern science becomes increasingly sophisticated and we are constantly bombarded with complicated information which is very often controversial. It is more and more difficult for the non-specialist to make value judgements in these important areas.

In order to follow the principles of holism it is necessary to gain as broad a picture as possible of all the things which have an influence on the life of the individual, whether environmental, physical or mental. These influences can then be assessed against health and well being. Holism may easily be put into practice given a basic working knowledge of relevant subjects, such as physiology and evolution.

The philosophy itself is sometimes thought of as somewhat mysterious, probably because some holistic medical practices are alien to our culture. Acupuncture is a good example. These practices often originated in Eastern cultures, and so were difficult to understand in relation to our own. Perseverance in trying to understand the principles of the therapies in our own terms has paid dividends in many therapeutic disciplines. Frequently the concept of a new therapy fits in with our established medicine once it is understood. The problem may simply be one of language.

In some cases, holistic therapies were established thousands of years ago. Many of them were initially dismissed as nonsense by modern science, and it is only comparatively recently that we have been able explain them in modern scientific terms.

The most rewarding approach by scientists is with an open mind: the willingness to have the flexibility to accept new and sometimes challenging ideas, when appropriate to do so. It was only through taking this approach that we have been able to explain, in our own scientific language, how some holistic therapies, such as acupuncture, work.

Holistic medicine such as homoeopathy is flourishing today, largely because of the side effects associated with modern pharmaceuticals or modern technological medicine. Holistic medicine uses substances which gently strengthen the innate powers of the body to overcome the problem. There is renewed interest in this concept as modern societies realise that there is more benefit in working with the natural order of things rather than against them.

It is commonly believed that 'alternative' medicines used as part of holistic therapy are ineffective in situations where heroic measures are required. This is a fallacy. Some holistic practitioners use alternative medicines almost to the exclusion of modern synthetic medicines. Indeed, many cases which are referred to holistic practitioners are successfully treated with alternative therapies where modern drug treatment has failed.

As with any new or, in this case, renewed interest involving principles and ideas which may be largely or partly misunderstood, there can be much confusion, and sometimes danger. There are many ill-conceived products, in particular herbal mixtures, being sold for horses which are formulated by unqualified individuals. Many of these are based on information which is extrapolated from human herbals. Not only is this practice irresponsible, it is also dangerous in some circumstances. Many such products contain ingredients which should not be used on a regular basis without veterinary advice, for example sedatives, analgesics, and substances which affect the hormonal system.

This only serves to throw the whole area into disrepute. Some holistic therapies involve the use of substances which can be very dangerous in the wrong hands. It is a common misconception that just because a substance is natural it is harmless. Curare, for example, is a natural substance but a deadly poison.

An example of one who suffered at the hands of ignorant people who meant well was Charles II, in 1685. Despite the fact that his physicians should arguably have been the best in the land, the king was prescribed medicines which are almost beyond belief. Lack of scientific knowledge and over-zealous use of various and potent substances by the physicians, no doubt in an attempt to gain royal patronage if the king recovered, probably killed him.

His treatment is well documented and is chronicled as follows by Christine Stockwell in her book, *Nature's pharmacy*:

On February 2nd 1685, whilst being shaved, the king was seized with a convulsion and collapsed, probably with a blood clot. First he was bled. An enema and two purgatives were administered, followed by an enema containing mallow leaves, violets, beetroot, camomile, fennel, linseed, cinnamon, cardamon, saffron and aloes – among other things. He was given snuff of powdered hellebore and another of cowslips. He was given, to drink, a mixture of barley water, liquorice and sweet almond, draughts of white wine, a cocktail of absinthe and anise and extracts of thistle leaves, mint, rue, angelica. Internal treatment continued with slippery elm, peony, lavender, lime flowers, lily of the valley, melon seeds and dissolved pearls. The physicians carried on their unholy assault with gentian root, nutmeg, quinine and cloves. They shaved the king's head and rubbed in powdered blistering beetles, meanwhile applying a drawing plaster of Burgundy pitch and pigeon droppings to his feet. They brought in Bezoar stones – perhaps thinking that he had been poisoned. None of this improved the king's condition even though a special dose of Raleigh's antidote was forced down his throat and, after four days, during which time he apologised for taking such 'an unconscionable time a-dying', the King died, surely with a sigh of relief.

The post-war sciences

In recent years many talented scientists have been attracted into the food and pharmaceutical manufacturing industries, and remarkable developments have taken place. Advanced chemical and biological sciences have provided many benefits for the modern consumer, and until very recently were seen to be the saviour of modern societies. Foods from foreign countries can be bought by most people, looking as fresh as the day they were gathered; flavours can be made in a laboratory; artificial colours can be added. Huge advances have also been made in all areas of medical science.

Many of these advances have been brought about largely because there is a market to justify the research. Food science and medical science are highly specialised and profitable businesses. Much of what is currently being developed, and has been developed over the last few decades, is market driven. There is a market for products which either try to fool the palate, or try to fool the body. In their enthusiasm to market such products the manufacturers have often allowed their belief in the positive aspects to overshadow or exclude attention to the negative aspects. Naturally the consumer has become disenchanted with the faith that was, perhaps unfairly, placed in modern science.

The twentieth century has seen leaps in science and technology that would have astounded our forebears. Along with new developments came the belief that everything can be explained in terms of modern science, and that there would be a scientific or technological answer to every problem. It became fashionable to dismiss the wisdom accrued over thousands of years as primitive and 'mumbo jumbo'. Modern man has placed too much faith in science.

There is no doubt that modern science has been beneficial to mankind, but we must keep a sense of perspective. It is a common misconception that medicine itself has been the largest contributor to the improvement of health in the twentieth century. In fact, although it has played an important part in treating the symptoms of disease, it has done little to prevent the cause. The largest contributor to the improvement of health was the public drainage system, which treated the cause of disease.

Modern medicine takes a compartmentalised approach to disease, usually treating symptoms with some invasive chemical agent. The holistic approach takes a broader view. Treatment consists of removing barriers to healing, and trusting in the body's vital energies to heal itself. Traditional medicine has taken this approach for thousands of years, and it is practised very successfully in many parts of the developed world.

Market forces

Many of the principles of selling human products, in terms of scientific knowledge, marketing pressures, attitudes and other issues, are now influencing the equine market. It is often said that changes in the veterinary market come ten years after those in the market for products for humans.

There are noticeably more products available for horses today which cater for the demand for 'green' manufacture. Issues about such things as preservatives, colours and raw material sources are beginning to receive attention, just as they did in the human market some years ago. We also see unnecessary backwaters of confusion, sometimes proliferated and exaggerated out of all proportion by those with a vested interest. Sensitive issues are made light of using modern sophisticated marketing techniques. While this does not apply to all manufacturers, the consumer should be aware of the potential pitfalls.

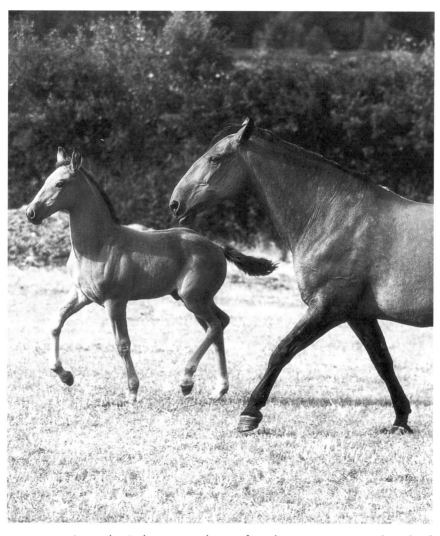

As mechanical power took over from horse power, many breeds of horse fell into decline. The Cleveland Bay, a traditional Yorkshire coaching horse, is now a rare breed.

Background to many of these issues will be given below in order that their importance may be considered by the reader wishing to put holistic principles into practice.

In evolutionary terms nothing has changed very much over the last few hundred years or so, so the basic biological needs and limitations of humans are exactly the same as they always were. The way we live in society today places great mental and physical strain on our bodies and we often forget that many ailments are a direct result of this. The biological sciences cannot make us into beings which can withstand these pressures. What they can usefully do is give us a deeper understanding of the nature of living beings. An holistic approach makes use of such knowledge, applying it in relation to the needs of the individual in modern society.

If we encounter problems when making value judgements for ourselves, what happens when we try to make them for horses? The same basic rules apply, of course. An unswerving dedication is needed to husbandry which takes into consideration the evolved requirements of the horse together with the effect that the act of domestication has on him.

In previous generations, those who undertook the daily management of animals, and did so efficiently and with the best interests of the animals at heart, developed a deep understanding of the animals in their care. They knew their animals from the inside out, and their knowledge was largely gained through experience – initially while under the guiding hand of a mentor – rather than through theoretical learning. They were called good stockmen if they were with farm animals, and good horsemen if they were responsible for horses. These terms were not applied lightly and those who were given the accolade received it with some pride.

The development of a thorough understanding of the horse is central to forming a realistic perspective on management practices. While the nature of the horse has not changed one iota since it was first domesticated, our treatment of it has changed because of a myriad of factors, with resultant effects on its health and welfare over the centuries.

In order to develop a balanced viewpoint and put the principles of holism into practice, an understanding of evolution, physiology, anatomy, behaviour and other associated subjects is useful. They may then be related to the management of the horse. Given an understanding of how these issues are intertwined and how they affect health and well-being, decisions can then be made regarding nutrition, farriery, exercise, grooming, tack and so on.

2

Man's relationship with the horse

'A horse misus'd upon the road Calls to Heaven for human blood.'
William Blake (1757–1827)

The horse as a 'symbol'

The horse occupies a place in the history of man unlike that of any other creature. He has been inextricably linked with man for many reasons, but up until recently the main one was the provision of a useful function. Until the development of mechanical power, animal-power was the only alternative to man-power, and this was usually provided by the horse. The different uses to which the horse has been put over generations is reflected in the many different types of horse we see today.

The basic conformation of the horse can be adapted for two main functions: his strength can be harnessed to operate machinery or to carry loads, and man can sit on his back and be carried. These two abilities have a variety of uses in the service of man, and a look at the purposes to which the horse has been put gives us a perspective on how it has developed under domestication. Developments usually involved breeding for specific conformation and temperament. Despite the very obvious differences which may be observed between certain breeds – the Shire and the Thoroughbred, for example – they are no thicker than a veneer, as we shall discuss later.

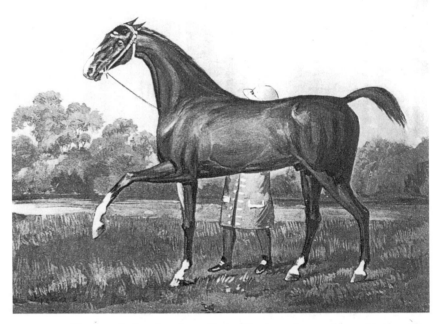

The popularity of racing reflected the importance of speed in the riding horse of the day. Flying Childers (foaled 1715), whose sire was the Darley Arabian, was reputedly the fastest horse ever over a long distance. If records are to be believed, at Newmarket he ran a distance of 3 miles, 6 furlongs and 93 yards in 6 minutes and 40 seconds. Even allowing for exaggeration it is fairly certain that he was the fastest horse of his day. (Detail from painting by Sartorius, after Seymour)

Apart from his usefulness to man, which of course has endeared the horse to us, there is the unfathomable relationship which flourishes despite the fact that we no longer depend upon horses as a source of power. This may be partially explained by the horse's influence as a powerful psychological 'symbol' for man.

The nature of symbolism and how it affects our lives is discussed by the eminent psychologist and philosopher Carl Jung in his book *Man and his symbols*. Through his work and writings, Jung was probably the first to describe the nature and importance of psychological symbols. He proposed that the part of the mind which is unconscious communicates with the conscious mind through symbolism. A healthy psyche is able to maintain the necessary balance between the two by integrating the messages contained in the symbols into everyday life. Interestingly, Jung also referred to

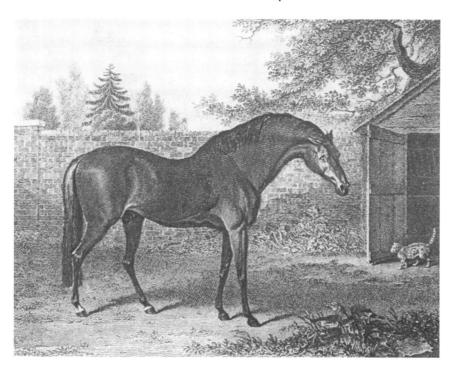

The Godolphin Arabian is one of the three founding sires of the Thoroughbred. He was imported into this country from France in 1728, apparently found between the shafts of a water cart in Paris, and he died in 1753. Legend has it that his companion cat (shown in the picture) disconsolately followed the horse to his grave and then mysteriously disappeared, never to be seen again.

the importance of 'wholeness', particularly with regard to the psyche.

Symbolism is an important part of life for many primitive societies, and Jung argued that they enjoy much better mental health because of it. Modern man tries to reduce the effect of this powerful phenomenon by using 'nothing but' explanations, which miss the point entirely. The use of modern 'scientific' explanations cannot remove the significance of symbols on the conscious mind, nor should it; it simply diverts the conscious mind temporarily. For example, we know that noise produced by thunder is 'nothing but' electrical activity, but this knowledge does not reduce its psychological impact for many people.

Symbols invoke emotions which are representative of inner workings of the psyche and they take many forms. They appear in all kinds of situations, such as dreams; there are also symbolic thoughts and feelings, symbolic acts and situations. The effects of a symbol on the conscious mind often defy rational explanation. Symbols are always more than they appear to be. For example, if asked why we like horse riding, we may say that we enjoy the exercise, the discipline, the companionship, the freedom; but all of these are conscious reasons, and, while they may be relevant, they skirt around the central point of the symbol. A more appropriate answer might be that we enjoy the 'feeling' of horse riding, rather than the sensations of it. The 'feeling' in this sense is invoked by the power of the symbol – it is raw and unfathomable. Symbolism is about emotions, and any attempt to explain it logically fails; the unconscious is, by definition, unknowable.

Examples of the symbolic power of the horse appear regularly in our culture. For example, Sewell's story of Black Beauty is much more than the simple tale it appears to be. Another example is the French film *Crin Blanc*, which tells the story of a boy who has developed a deep friendship with a wild white stallion which still runs with its herd. While riding the stallion the boy is pursued by a group of horsemen who are rounding up wild horses for their own ends. After a long chase, the horse and the boy are eventually caught between the horsemen and the sea. Rather than be captured, they plunge into the sea and are swept away.

Time and time again this symbolism appears in stories through the ages and it is just as powerful today, finding its way into many areas of modern society. For example, it is used by the advertising industry for commercial ends. One of the national banks used it to imprint their image on the minds of television viewers, many of whom presumably are not horse-owners, or who may not have even seen a horse in the flesh. The emotions stirred by the image of the galloping black horse to a background of powerful music are obviously not limited to horse riders: this is a universal symbol in the 'Jungian' sense of the word.

There have been many stories over the centuries of man's unique relationship with the horse. These stories are often about military leaders, for whom the horse has special importance. On horseback they could quickly cover the field of battle, and they could easily be seen by other members of the group. One example of this is Alexander's well-documented love for his horse Bucephalus; another, Cyrus' for his favourite horse, which was drowned beneath

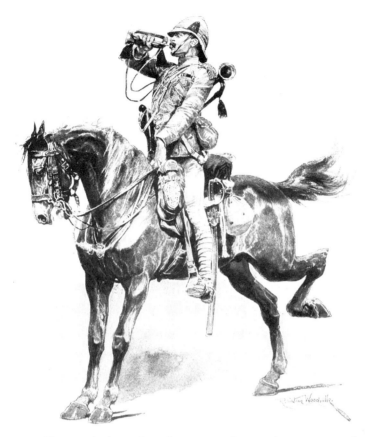

The cavalry horse in action was much more than a means of transport; he also inspired resolution and courage. Even though, thankfully, he has no place in war today, this important role continues in ceremonial duties.

him as he attempted to traverse the flooded river Diyala, in Mesopotamia. So distraught was Cyrus that as a revenge he is said to have had his army divert the river into many segments, so that it ran into the desert and died. Typical of these stories is that the owner of such animals was often a leader, and usually in a privileged or wealthy position; they certainly all shared an uncompromising passion for their horses.

The use of the horse in military service no doubt inspired a sense of duty towards him like no other, and even though the horse has little place in war today, his use in associated ceremonial duties continues. The funeral cortège of someone who achieves high military rank still includes his charger, complete with his empty boots strapped backwards into the stirrups. There is also a tradition in one mounted regiment where a charger is ridden up the main steps of a church, and stands in the building for the duration of the service.

The horse has always been associated, in many other cultures as well as our own, with freedom, power, dominion, and libido. The reasons for this may appear to be obvious, but there is a far deeper significance, as we have seen. The horse has religious associations in some cultures; his place in mythology and his relationship with the unicorn and the centaur also illustrate his importance as a symbol. A Greek legend, for example, tells the story of Chiron the centaur, half man and half horse, who possessed great knowledge of herbs and medicine and was worshipped as a god.

There are many superstitions associated with horse-shoes. They were thought to keep evil spirits away, because their shape was incompatible with the cloven foot of the 'evil one', and they were similar in shape to the halos around the heads of saints and angels in ancient religious pictures. They were also thought to have been 'purified', having been passed through fire. If horses were suffering from some kind of ailment that the farrier did not understand, this was commonly attributed to witchcraft, and a cure was attempted by removing the shoes and placing them in the fire again to drive out the spell.

Farmers of the eighteenth century believed that milk could be bewitched (*The Farmer's Magazine*). They thought that this was why at certain times of the year it was more difficult to make butter from the milk, and in order to drive out the devil a red-hot horse-shoe was plunged into the milk. Horse-shoes were commonly nailed on to the cow houses for protection. Sailors of the same time commonly nailed a horse-shoe to the mizzen mast, or somewhere on deck near mid-ships for the protection of the vessel.

A report in 1832 (*The Farmer's Magazine*) refers to information from a Captain Hall, who noted that the Chinese had their tombs built in the shape of the horse-shoe. This was thought to be very curious at the time because it was considered that such superstitions were only prevalent amongst the British.

Horse brasses were also used to keep evil spirits away, being fastened to the harness. Like the horse-shoe, they continue to be used to bring good luck.

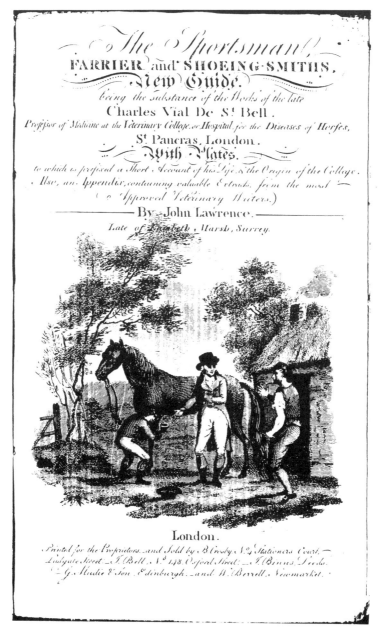

The frontispiece of *Farrier and shoeing-smiths* (1796), a collection of extracts from 'approved veterinary writers' of the day. It also gives an account of the origins of the veterinary college at St Pancras, London. It was not until 85 years later, in 1881, that the Veterinary Surgeons Act required the college to maintain and publish a register of veterinary surgeons.

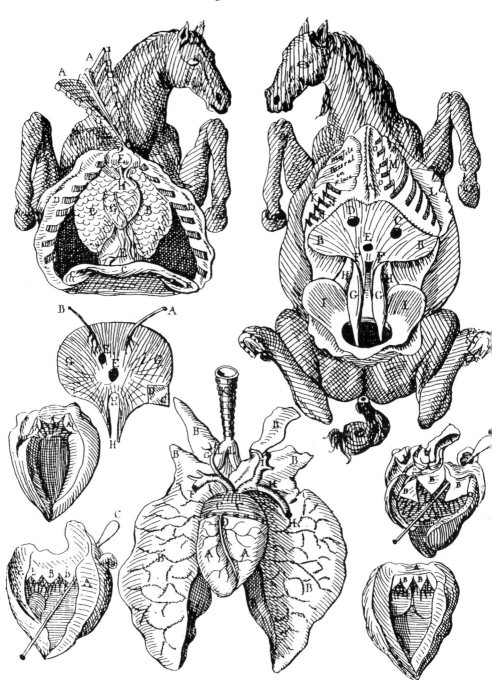

General anatomy of the horse as understood 250 years ago. Reproduced from anatomical plates, Garsault, *L'Anatomie générale du cheval*, 1734.

Evolving attitudes

Up until the mid to late eighteenth century our general attitude towards animals was backward by modern standards. Although we had progressed, thankfully, from the dark ages, when animals were actually tried and, if found guilty, executed for their crimes, we still behaved towards them with little compassion. During those times the streets of most towns would be filled with animals of all descriptions: horses and other beasts of burden would haul their miserable loads under curses and beatings, herds of animals from the country would be arriving, driven on foot to the slaughter-houses, exhausted and suffering from the effects of the journey. Popular pastimes of the day included bull-baiting, dog-fighting, and cock-fighting. Most people were apathetic towards the suffering of animals, and in fact it was probably regarded as a healthy attitude to posses a lust for giving them a hard time.

Life in those days was very harsh by our standards and this probably accounted for the way in which animals were treated generally. If humans had to suffer, why should animals be treated any better? It was commonly felt that animals had no soul. They were thought of as automatons, which probably helped people to absolve themselves of blame for their plight.

In 1800, a Bill was presented to Parliament with the intention of abolishing bull-baiting. So uninterested were most members that few turned up, and after some debate, the Bill was rejected. During the well-documented discussions on the Bill, the future prime minister, George Canning, defended bull-baiting. He said that 'the amusement inspired courage, and produced a nobleness of sentiment and elevation of the mind' (Manning & Serpell, *Animals and human society*).

No doubt the horse suffered at the hands of the masses in those times, no less than other animals. This brings the reputation of the British as animal lovers into historical perspective. But there is some evidence that general attitudes towards horses were gradually becoming more humane during the first half of the nineteenth century. The editor of the *The Farmer's Magazine*, a periodical

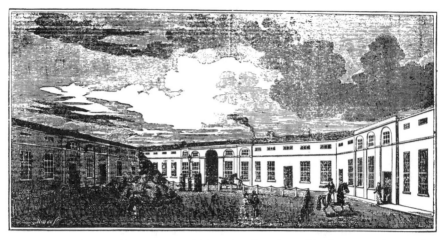

The Royal Veterinary College London, from *The farrier and naturalist,* Zoological Society of London, 1828. Whilst the 'veterinary art' has been studied since man was first associated with animals, formal education increased as veterinary science progressed. Although general attitudes towards animals gradually became more humane during the first half of the nineteenth century, a few years before this engraving was completed a bill to abolish bull-baiting in England was rejected by Parliament.

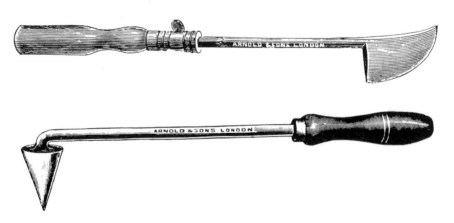

Firing is a very old practice going back several centuries. It involved hot irons being applied to the horse's legs as a treatment for lameness. Although there was more general use of chloroform at the beginning of the twentieth century, firing was of concern to veterinarians and owners on humane grounds. The practice began to decline, and today it is no longer recommended by the veterinary profession.

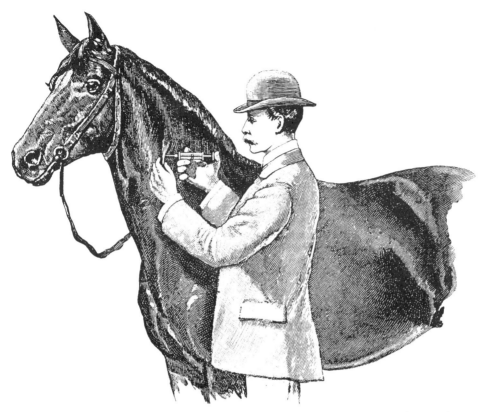

The veterinary surgeon, *c.* 1900. During the Victorian age, the rapid advancement of veterinary science meant that standards of health care improved dramatically.

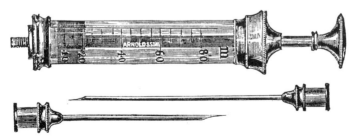

Late Victorian hypodermic syringe and needles. These were engineered to a very high standard so they would withstand the rigours of regular use and sterilising by heat or chemicals. With the increasing use of injectable pharmaceutical medicines and the advent of mass-produced, single use, sterile plastic syringes and needles, these handsome precision instruments became obsolete.

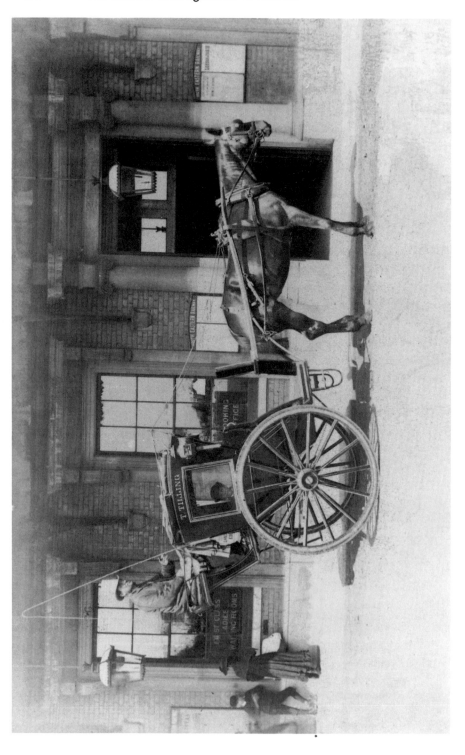

newspaper, wrote on Friday 17 August 1832:

Then if the horse be thus ready to exert himself for our pleasure, and pleasure alone is here the object, it is indefensible and brutal to urge him beyond his natural ardour, so severely as we sometimes do, and even until nature is quite exhausted. We do not often hear of a 'hard day' [hunting], without being likewise informed that one or more horses either died in the field or scarcely reached home before they expired. Some have been thoughtless and cruel enough to kill two horses in one day. One of the severest chases on record was by the king's stag hounds. There was an uninterrupted burst of four hours and twenty minutes. One horse dropped dead in the field, another died before he could reach the stable and seven more within a week after.

After several paragraphs of further references to 'merciless riders', the editor goes on to describe the symptoms of exhaustion, and concludes: 'The man who proceeds a single mile after this, ought to suffer the punishment he is inflicting.' Strong words indeed, considering the harder sentiments prevailing at the time.

While things were certainly improving, the generally poor treatment of animals continued more or less up until the middle of the nineteenth century. The real change in our attitudes towards animals came in the Victorian age (Manning & Serpell, *Animals and human society*). It emanated from the high morals of the society at the time, and was led by Queen Victoria herself who, along with many members of her court, became patrons of several animal welfare movements. There began to be a general improvement in the way that all animals were treated.

Along with this came the new biological sciences, and a great deal was learned about the horse and other animals during that time. Because of his importance as a source of power and transport at home, and also throughout the vast Victorian empire, there was

(Opposite) Horses such as these rarely, if ever, had the pleasure of being turned out to grass. They had to earn their keep nearly every day of their working life. The hansom cab was a common form of transport for one or two people in most cities until the introduction of the motor car. The burden on the horse could be eased by the driver who adjusted his position to compensate for the weight of the passengers. The small boy inside this hansom cab waiting outside a London railway station in 1885 has probably jumped aboard for the benefit of the photographer, as no self-respecting driver would have driven off with the shafts in the air throwing the cab hopelessly out of balance.

a financial incentive to make use of the new sciences in improving the health and welfare of the horse.

During this period knowledge and standards of veterinary care, feeding and general management improved at an unprecedented rate. The accumulated knowledge of the various scientific disciplines was being published as never before. While there were many books published on horses previously, those produced during the Victorian age were far more comprehensive. They were able to reflect on the established practices of equestrianism in the light of knowledge gained through the new sciences.

Despite the accumulation of knowledge during the Victorian age there are many practices we would reject today on humanitarian grounds. Many of these were carried out because the horse was fundamentally a working animal providing a service for man. Horses were often subjected to severe training methods and conditions, which naturally caused some animals to become vicious and unmanageable. Undoubtedly the best horsemen were successful because they were able to combine the benefits of the new 'sciences' with their skill and knowledge of the horse. This was only possible because of their close relationship with them.

The development of a 'market'

The way in which we treat animals may be directly related to the financial association we have with them. Even after the changes which took place in Victorian times the farmer still had to take a detached view of the animals in his care. As commercial pressures on agriculture grew, livestock farming became more intensive; and although certain of these methods are falling out of favour today, we developed sophisticated scientific methods of production to increase output.

Intensive livestock production is possible in part because of improvements in management, such as attention to hygiene. However, the largest commercial advantages are be to gained by the artificial manipulation of the animals' natural physiology. Apart from the moral issues involved, there are numerous disadvantages, particularly with regard to health and welfare, which will be discussed later.

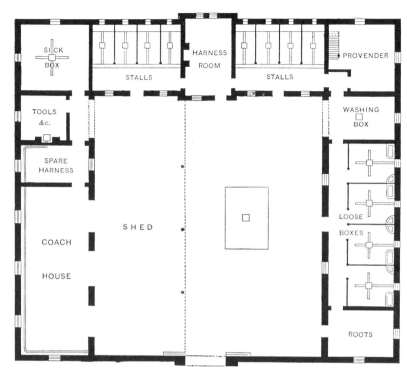

Plan of early Victorian stable buildings for twelve horses. The frequent use of stalls often made horses irritable, leading to vices and sometimes viciousness in the hands of unsympathetic grooms.

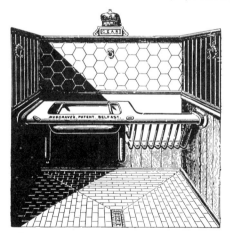

Consideration for well-designed equipment is illustrated by this early Victorian manger and hay-rack. Nothing can easily injure the horse and there is nothing which a mischievous animal could easily damage. Easily cleaned surfaces and minimum waste of food are also of prime importance.

The science which enabled these practices of husbandry to operate was developed because of commercial pressure. Because the need was there, and the new biological sciences were able to fill that need, a huge and profitable market developed, gaining momentum from about the middle of the twentieth century to the present day. Many products, such as vaccines and artificial vitamins, were developed largely because there was a financial incentive. Their development is extremely costly and could only be justified by rewards in the market place.

The financial incentive existed not only to develop pharmaceutical products to combat disease, but also to develop feeds which were designed to improve food conversion ratios. These skills were often developed at the expense of the health and welfare of the animals concerned. Many longer-term problems associated with the use of some products are only just coming to light.

At the other end of the animal scale, there was also a commercial incentive to develop products for animals kept as domestic pets, such as the cat and the dog. A need grew for vaccines to combat diseases caused by urban overcrowding. There was also a need for convenience foods for the busy modern owner. As with the products developed for agricultural species, there were underlying physiological and philosophical concerns which we are only now beginning to focus on.

The equine market was partially ignored in this scientific development. There was little financial incentive until recently to justify the same amount of research. Even when the boom in equestrianism as a leisure pursuit came, many products, including pharmaceutical products and feeding stuffs for horses, began to be developed and sold on the basis of research on other species. This was done largely as a short-cut, and it is a flawed approach carrying health risks. In the light of the health problems we are now seeing as a result of this practice, we rightly question some of these principles.

As with other species, the demand for horse products was brought about by changes in management practices. There was a greater need to develop methods to control disease, largely caused by increased numbers of horses in concentrated areas, as with domestic pets; also the busy modern horse-owner, like the pet owner, required feeding stuffs as a ready mixed product. The equestrian market has developed rapidly since the 1970s.

It is becoming increasingly difficult to maintain a balanced view of horse management. As well as the continuing changes in farming methods which affect the horse, there is the unrelenting pressure from manufacturers to entice the horse-owner to purchase particular brands, often on the pretext of some 'discovery' or other. Nutrition is a good example of this. Feeding horses need not be complicated provided the basic rules are followed; that is, the exclusive use of raw materials which are closest to horses' evolved requirements. The myth that horses must be fed according to the 'modern scientific' approach is largely perpetuated by the feed industry itself, which is usually trying to justify the use of unsuitable raw materials. This leads to unnecessary confusion, and the often unwitting use of ingredients which would not otherwise be used by the horse owner.

The principles of good management hold, whatever the species, and will go a long way to promote health and fitness. We have already said that the management of the horse as practised by our Victorian forefathers was superior in many ways to that of today. But we have seen that we must balance our approach between the attitudes which prevailed then, and our own requirements and knowledge in this 'enlightened' age. It is within this framework that we can begin to examine the principles and practice of holistic management.

The attitude of the farmer has always been pragmatic, developed out of necessity rather than cold-heartedness. When times are hard the commercial facts of life mean that animals have to earn their keep. The horse was no exception to this rule. Man's relationship with the horse, as well as with other farm animals, has probably changed more in the twentieth century than in any other. The main change has been in our attitude. We now see animals, including the horse, in a different light, largely unfettered by the preconceptions that using them for a particular purpose brought about.

The change in the general attitude towards the keeping of farm animals has been largely a result of consumer action. The trend is to keep animals in conditions which are more extensive, which has a direct influence on health. In looking at the changes which have occurred we can chart the relationship between how animals are kept and treated and the development of various diseases. We can also see how modern science has attempted to defeat such diseases by the use of increasingly desperate methods, such as bombarding livestock with numerous vaccines.

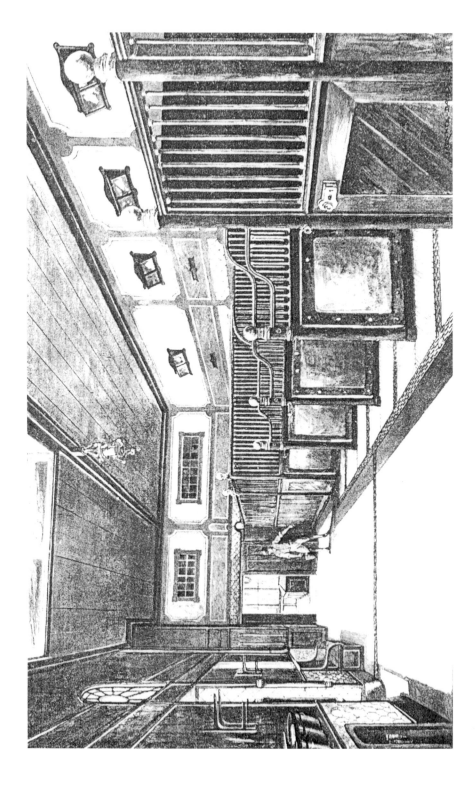

Domestication and health

The cause of most of the diseases and ailments of the animals in our care is directly related to the conditions in which they are kept. Domestication involves compromises in many areas, and although it is an over-simplification to say that animals in the wild are rarely ill, it illustrates the point.

Any human modifications on behavioural, environmental and nutritional aspects of the species carry a risk. The risk is a matter of degree, but it is none the less a risk. The compromises which domestication forces upon us with regard to any one of these factors will have a negative effect on the health and well-being of the animal. It follows that the less we interfere with the natural order of things, the fewer health problems will arise. The essence of holistic management is to reduce these compromises so that their effects are acceptable.

An example of this is the common farmyard hen, whose 'health programme' probably consists of no more than periodic cleaning of the hen house, and occasional dusting with 'louse powder'. She will probably live quite happily for a number of years, pecking around for this and that, in conditions which are mostly conducive to good health and a sense of well-being.

Intensive egg-farming is an entirely different matter. It involves cramming four laying hens into a small cage, in which they can barely turn around – for life. Their food is largely made from by-products, probably including some of their own dried droppings liberally laced with drugs of one sort or other, and they are probably killed after one year, because their egg production drops. Many suffer from congenital defects, brought about by intensive breeding, and some are almost featherless through aggressive pecking caused by overcrowding. Their musculo-skeletal system breaks down as a result of confinement. They are not referred to

(Opposite) As science began to explain the way diseases spread, high standards of cleanliness in stable management became paramount in Victorian stables. The importance of the horse as a working animal justified the substantial expense involved in buildings of this type, which was reflected in the superb craftsmanship of the day.

WALES HALL

WALES, Near Sheffield.

1½ miles from Kiveton Park and 1 mile from Waleswood G.C. Station.
Sheffield to Anston Buses pass the Farm.

CATALOGUE

OF THE WHOLE OF THE

LIVE and DEAD FARMING-STOCK,

comprising:

HARNESS,
IMPLEMENTS,
SMALL TOOLS,
86 SHEEP,
55 BEAST,
15 HORSES,
7 PIGS,
POULTRY,
PRODUCE,
DAIRY UTENSILS,

ETC.

W. T. PARKER

favoured with instructions from Mr. A. GREAVES (who is retiring), will SELL BY AUCTION, on

MONDAY, MARCH 13th, 1922.

SALE TO COMMENCE AT 11 A.M.

Refreshments may be obtained near the Premises.

	£	s.	d.

14 Black Yearling Colt, out of "Daisy"
15 Brown Yearling Colt; out of "Violet."

PIGS.

2 Strong Stores
2 ditto
2 ditto
1 ditto

POULTRY.

10 couples Fowls

PRODUCE.

Cob Wheat Straw
Ditto
Ditto
Ditto

DAIRY UTENSILS.

Bradford's End-over-End Churn, to Churn 20 lbs.
Butter Worker
Milk Buckets
Scyle
Measures
Cheese Pan
Stilton Cheese Hoops
Diabolo No. 1 Separator in very good order.

SPORTING DOG.

Black and White Spaniel Dog, broken to Gun.

	£	s.	d.

26 Black Ditto
27 Red Heifer served for Aug. 26th
28 Roan Heifer served for Aug. 12th
29 Roan Heifer served for July 4th
30 Red and White Bullock
31 Black ditto, 18 months
32 2 Red Heifers
33 2 Red and White ditto, 18 months
34 2 Ditto
35 2 Ditto
36 Fat Bull Calf (suckling on cow)
37 Rearing Bull 6 months
38 Rearing Bull, 6 months
39 2 Heifer Calves, 8 months
40 2 Ditto
41 2 Ditto
42 2 Steers, 8 months
43 2 Heifer Calves, 3 months
44 2 Bull Calves, 3 months
45 Calf, 2 months

15 HORSES.

1 Roan Clydesdale Mare "Kitty," rising 5 years, 16 h.h., sire "Wreay Viceroy," believed in foal to "Mallow Drayman"
2 Black Clydesdale Mare, "Darkie," rising 5 years, 17 h.h., eligible for Stud Book, sire "Craigie Captain, 17859"
3 Brown Mare "Daisy," by Scarcliffe Manners"
4 Chestnut Mare, 16 h.h., "Violet," by "Scarcliffe Manners"
5 Brown Mare "Bonnie," rising 4 years, by "German William," quiet and good worker
6 Brown half-legged Horse "Bob"
7 Black Mare, "Diamond," quiet and a good worker
8 Brown Filly, rising 2 years, by "Scarcliffe Friarlike"
9 Black Gelding, rising 2 years, by "Scarcliffe Friarlike,"
10 Brown Filly, rising 2 years
11 Brown Gelding, rising 2 years
12 Brown half-legged Filly, rising 2 years
13 Brown Yearling Colt, out of Clydesdale Mare, "Darkie"

CATALOGUE.

—o—

HARNESS and TACKLING.

4 Sets Cart Harness, complete
2 Sets Sling Gears
3 pairs of Plough Pads
Set of silver-plated Trap Harness
Set of Float Harness
Breast Collar
Set of Breaking Tackle
5 Head Collars
Pair Pole Straps
Extra Collars and Bluffs
Stable Utensils
Horse Clipping Machine

IMPLEMENTS & SMALL TOOLS.

Hay Rakes and Forks
Dung Forks and Shovels
Thatch Pegs
Cart Ropes
Pair Wheels and Axle
2 Sheep Troughs
2 ditto
2 ditto
2 ditto
Sheep Cratch on wheels
Knife Stand
Metal Pig Trough
Corn Bins
Mixing Tubs
Large Zinc Water Tank
Wood Tumbril
Hay Knife
Wheel Barrow, new
Joiners' Bench
Ladder
Ditto
New ditto, 32 staves
Whitewashing Machine
Set of Pulleys and chain to lift 1 ton
Picker Pole
New-sawn Timber
Sheep Netting
Sack Lifter
Avery Platform Weighing Machine

Cake Breaker
Hay Knife
Burman's Sheep Clipping Machine
3-horse Iron Drag
Massey-Harris Spring Tyne Cultivator
International Harvesting Co. Ditto
Martin's 7-Tyne Cultivator
Horse Hoe
Ditto
Roberts' Ditto
Ransome Digger
Plough with Ridging Breast
Cooke's Plough, R.U.S. 9; with digger breast
Cooke's X.L. 2 Plough
Cooke's X.L.S.S. Ditto
Set of 3 Iron Harrows
Set of 2 Ditto
Set of 3 Turnip Harrows
Stone Roller with metal frame
4-Cylinder Metal Flat Roller
Cambridge Roller, new
Yates' Turnip Drill with side hoes
Massey-Harris Disc Drill
Albion Grass Mower, new
Wood's Grass Mower
Massey-Harris Binder in good order
Blackstone Swath Turner
Horse Rake
Bamford's Ditto
Set of Chain Harrows
Manco Petrol Engine, $1\frac{1}{2}$ h.p.
Belting
Bamford's Pulper, hand or power
Hay Wagon in good order
Heavy Cart, nearly new
Heavy Cart with Shelvings and Gormers, in good order
Ditto
Ditto
Ditto
Milk Float
4-wheel Dog Cart with Rubber Tyres
Dog Cart, nearly new, by Stacey, Nottingham

86 SHEEP.

1 5 Strong Cross-bred in-lamb Ewes and Lambs
2 5 Strong Cross-bred in-lamb Ewes and Lambs
3 5 ditto
4 5 ditto
5 5 ditto
6 5 ditto
7 5 ditto
8 5 ditto
9 5 ditto
10 2 ditto
11 5 Fat Hogs
12 5 ditto
13 5 ditto
14 5 ditto
15 5 ditto
16 5 ditto
17 5 ditto
18 4 ditto

55 BEAST.

1 Red Lincoln Bull, $2\frac{1}{2}$ yrs.
2 Roan Cow, 3rd note, served for May 3rd
3 Red and White Cow served for 19th June
4 Ditto for Sept. 1st
5 Red Cow, barren, in milk
6 Red and White Cow in full milk
7 Red and White Cow, pasture served
8 Red Heifer in full milk, barren
9 Red Ditto
10 Roan Ditto
11 Roan Heifer
12 Red and White Cow, 3rd note, pasture served
13 Red Cow, 2nd note at hand
14 Red Heifer, pasture served
15 Ditto
16 Red and White Ditto
17 Ditto
18 Red Bullock in forward condition
19 Ditto
20 Ditto
21 Ditto
22 Roan Poll Heifer, served for 26th May
23 Roan Heifer, pasture served
24 Red and White Ditto
25 Ditto

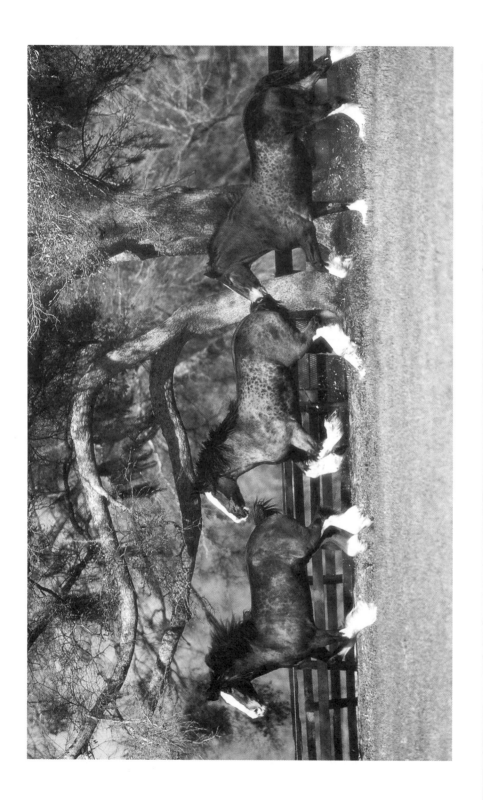

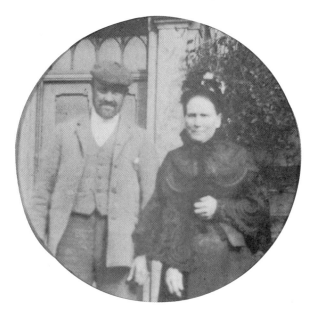

Mr and Mrs A. Greaves of Wales Hall, Chesterfield (see farm sale catalogue). Mr Greaves was born in the 1850s and during his lifetime the horse was the central source of power in agriculture, as it had been for countless generations before. The development of the internal combustion engine some eighty years later changed forever the role of the horse, not only in farming, but in almost every other sphere.

(Previous pages) Farm auction sale catalogue, 1922. The former relationship between man and the horse in farming life may be appreciated from this list of the entire contents of the farm, which provides an interesting 'snapshot'. As well as operating the wide range of farm implements, wagons and machinery, horses would have been used to transport the family between the shafts of the dog-cart, and also to deliver milk to the local trader. The listings in the catalogue give an indication of the relative importance of the horse at the time: all the horses are named, but the other animals (including the dog!) are not, even though the milking cows and bulls would almost certainly have had names, as they do today.

(Opposite) The magnificent Shire. Before the development of tractors, gentle giants such as these provided ample power for heavy agricultural work such as ploughing. In some situations they are capable of working land that is inaccessible to their mechanical successors, and Heavy Horse Societies ensure the continuation of the breeds.

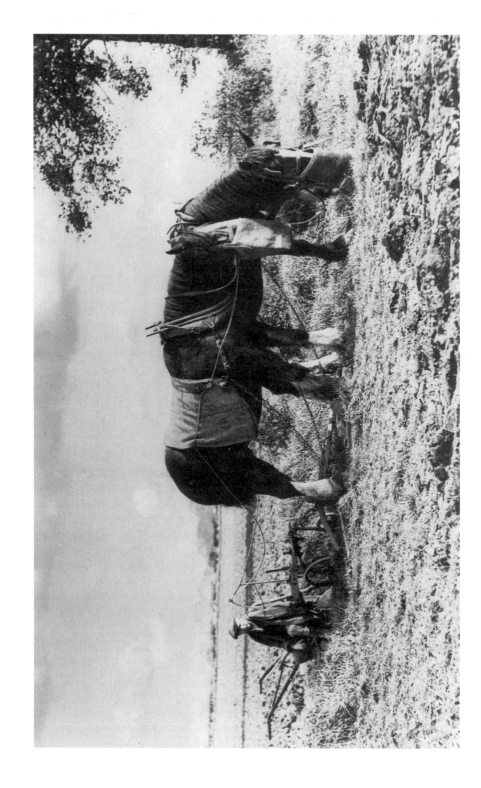

as flocks of hens, but crops. This type of management forces the use of vaccines against at least five different diseases, some having to be sprayed into the atmosphere every three weeks or so. The incidence of disease is directly related to the degree of intensification. Spread the population out and there are fewer problems crowd them and there are more. Many would now agree that the compromises involved here to the health and welfare of both the hens and the consumer are not outweighed by the production of cheap eggs.

This approach to egg production is taken for commercial reasons, and although an extreme example it illustrates the pragmatic attitude which has prevailed in farming for many generations. Although, generally, the methods used could not be said to be cruel in the true sense of the word, many modern consumers would say that the methods involved are not acceptable if there is an alternative. Their counterparts a generation or two before would have seen it as an undesirable but necessary method of producing cheap eggs. Today there are many alternative food sources available, and we do not have to use the products of intensive livestock systems if we disapprove of them.

So domestication is a compromise. We cannot help but have an influence on the potential for health problems arising, but what we can do is reduce the risks to a more acceptable level. Commercial production involving animals is being reviewed, and generally there is a trend away from intensive farming. This has happened as a concession towards modern sensibilities concerning animal welfare, and also because of fears concerning human health. Pressure is on farmers to use methods which are healthier both for the animals and for the consumer.

This background, and the reasons behind our general attitude towards animals, is relevant when considering the horse. In agriculture, the horse was essentially a source of power, and was regarded rather like a tractor would be today. When he outlived

(Opposite) 'Two horsepower.' Whilst the design of ploughs and other farm implements was improved as better materials for their construction became available, the basic concept had not changed for generations. The power of the horse was central to the annual task of turning the soil for seeding next year's crops. In this photograph taken during the early years of the twentieth century the ploughman gives his horses (and probably himself) a mid-day meal and a well-earned rest.

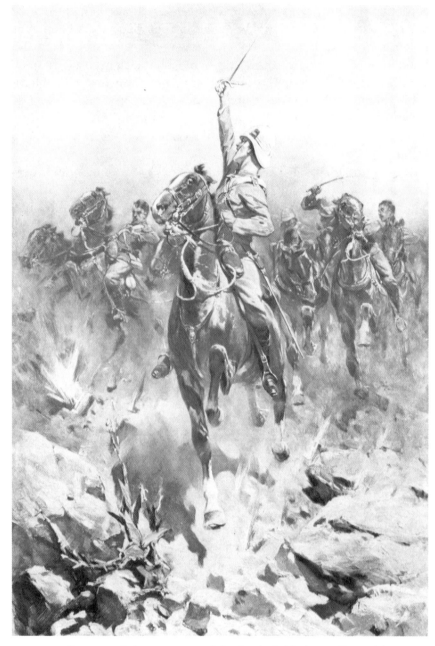

Because of the pressures of the battle-field, the welfare of horses in action was secondary to the waging of battle. In modern competition sports such as eventing, which has close links with traditional military training, the welfare of the horse can and should be put first. The competitor may honourably retire if necessary.

his economic usefulness, his fate was in the lap of the gods. To take any other approach could have risked the financial integrity of the farm. It was a business like any other, and there were no alternatives for most ordinary farmers. Despite the fact that the farmer must have had a particularly close relationship with the horse, feelings often had to be put aside in the light of agricultural necessity.

These attitudes were reflected in the way that the horse was treated generally. Most management systems were designed to produce the most work from the animal. Fortunately for the horse, good health and well-being were conducive to efficient work. Benefits were to be had by giving the horse a good diet and looking after his general welfare. However, when the horse became ill the main purpose of the treatment was to get him back to work as soon as possible, which sometimes involved the use of unkind and often cruel practices. There were many approaches to the treatment of injured or sick horses that we would find unacceptable today, largely because we have a choice.

Horses in Britain today are mainly treated as companion animals, rather than solely as an adjunct to work. The fact that most horses are now used mainly for recreation has two important consequences which relate to the principles of modern management and health care.

First, because we have the choice, we can reduce the potential for problems associated with over-exertion. An example of this is how we approach fitness and 'work', in the modern use of the expression. For instance, three-day eventing, particularly at advanced level, involves feats of Herculean proportions. In human terms, at the highest level of competition, the horse's fitness can be compared to an Olympic triathlon competitor. Eventing started as a competition for cavalry horses, essentially as a gauge of their potential in battle. The training and capability of the horse were vital to the effectiveness and survival of his rider. Because of these priorities training was essentially harsh, designed to reflect battle conditions, and accidents which occurred in those circumstances were seen as incidental and of secondary importance. Today the sport is governed by strict rules to minimise the potential for accidents, and those taking part are not under external pressure to take unnecessary risks which may endanger the horse. They can withdraw; this was not an option for a cavalry-man during battle.

Also they can indulge in a gradual build-up to fitness.

On the other hand, there are those whose desire to win is so overwhelming that they are not above using methods which would be condemned as cruel by compassionate people. Unfortunately this attitude is quite common, and either stems from financial reward in the form of prize money or sponsorship, or simply from the selfish motives of the rider or owner. This happens in all sections of the equestrian world, and is generally frowned upon as an unsporting and unhealthy attitude. The true horseman and horsewoman will put the health and well-being of the horse far above winning any competition, no matter what the rewards are.

In general the modern owner can be much more relaxed about performance; if the horse does not excel at a certain discipline he can concentrate on another. There are changing attitudes concerning the morality of the high-risk equine activities, such as racing, which are doing a great deal to reduce the risks in some sports. Today it is accepted that the horse does not have to be 'used' for anything. Many take great pleasure from plodding down a country lane on a favourite companion. Others keep horses simply for the pleasure of their company, and never ride. Horses nowadays are not regarded as 'useless' if they are unable to work, as they would have been by previous generations, since they no longer have to earn their keep. These are new, more humane, and certainly more compassionate times with regard to the treatment of horses.

The second consequence of the horse's mainly recreational use, again because there is in theory no great pressure to return to work, is that the types of therapy used in the treatment of various ailments can be far more relaxed and in tune with the body's own healing process. Most modern as well as some traditional methods of treating agricultural animals have an aspect of urgency prompted by finance which may influence the choice of treatment given. In the holistic approach, which does not involve this pressure so directly, alternative methods may be used. Many of these were in fact used before the advent of modern pharmaceutical drugs; with familiarity we may be surprised at how quickly they work.

3

Evolution and tradition

1 handful Wormwood
1 handful Rue
1 handful Rosemary
1 handful Box
1 oz. Tobacco
1 gallon Chamberlie [human urine]
Early-twentieth-century recipe for a 'bad feeder', used to wet the ration.

The evolution of the horse

The basic requirement of holistic nutrition is the use of raw materials which are as close as possible to those which the horse has evolved to eat. Examining the evolution of the modern horse helps us to understand its needs in the context of modern domestication. The horse was domesticated a mere 5,000 years ago, and although it has been adapted by man, to a certain extent, through breeding for conformation and temperament, this is only a thin veneer. There has been little time in evolutionary terms for horses to change.

The earliest relative of the horse, the forerunner of the modern counterpart, was Eohippus, the dawn horse. He existed about 55 million years ago, pre-dating man by more than 50 million years. He was about the size of a fox terrier and had four toes on each front foot and three on each hind foot. His habitat was semi-forest areas where he lived on a varied diet, including soft fruits and berries. His size and shape meant that he was ideally suited to this environment. A plentiful diet was within easy reach, and he had abundant cover in which to evade predators.

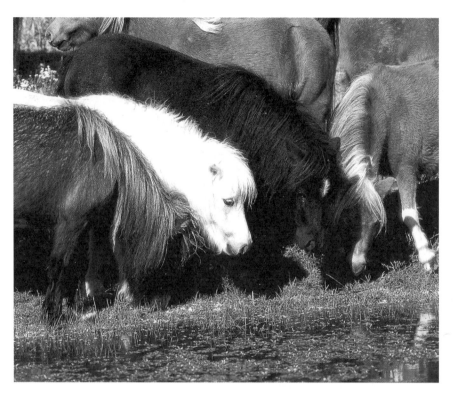

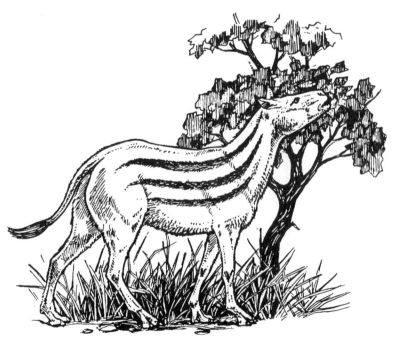

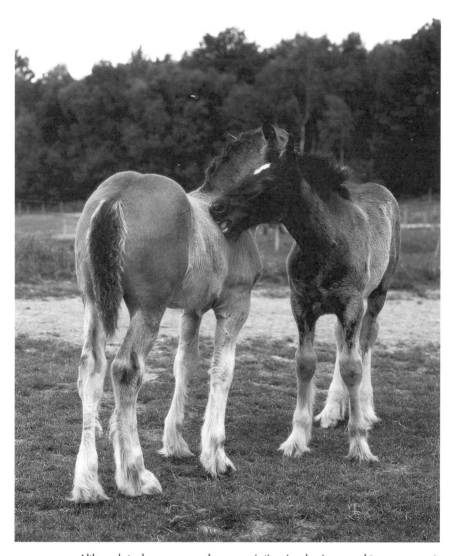

Although today we see a large variation in physique and temperament, the horse is little different from the wild creature that was domesticated 5000 years ago. Although these miniature horses (top left) are only a fraction of the size of the Shire horse foals (right) their basic physiology is the same.

(Left) Eohippus was probably the first true horse. He was about the size of a fox and lived on marshy ground. He had splayed toes and ate a wide variety of herbage and fruits.

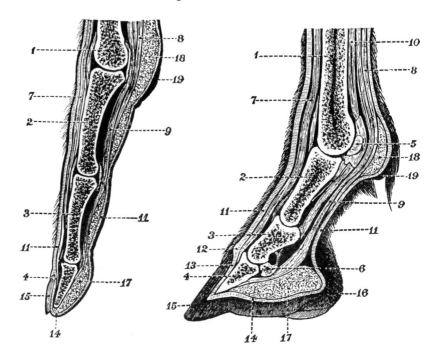

1. Metacarpal bone.
2. First phalanx.
3. Second phalanx.
4. Third phalanx (pedal bone of horse).
(5–6 wanting).
7. Tendon of extensor muscles.
8. Tendon of superficial flexor.
9. Tendon of deep flexor.
11 and 14. Derma or true skin.
15. Nail (imperfect hoof of horse).
17. Fibro-fatty cushion of end of finger.
18. Fibro-fatty cushion of palm behind metacarpal phalangeal joint.
19. Thickened epidermal covering of the same.

1. Metacarpal bone.
2. First phalanx.
3. Second phalanx.
4. Third phalanx.
5. One of the upper sesamoid bones.
6. Lower sesamoid or navicular bone.
7. Tendon of extensor muscle.
8. Tendon of superficial flexor.
9. Tendon of deep flexor.
10. Short flexor or suspensory ligament of the fetlock.
11. Derma or true skin continued into
12. Coronary cushion.
13, 14. Villous portion of the hoof matrix.
15. Hoof.
16. The heel.
17. Plantar cushion.
18. Fibro-fatty cushion of the fetlock.
19. Horny excrescence or spur (ergot).

Sections of finger of man and foot of horse. The horse walks on a modified third digit. This illustration shows the surviving similarities between the structures which have been adapted for very different purposes.

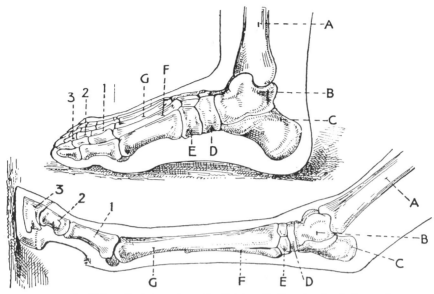

A, Tibia. B, Astragalus. C, Calcis. D, Scaphoid. E, Internal
cuneiform. F, Splint-bone (a vestige of 2nd metatarsal). G, Cannon
bone, or 3rd metatarsal. 1, 2, 3, Phalanges.

Foot of man and horse in their 'natural' positions. The similarities
between the two may be seen by comparing the bone structures. The
different mechanical stresses suffered in each case will be appreciated
by comparing the weight-bearing surfaces.

The species slowly moved out into the open plains, and this
meant very gradual changes of anatomy. Less cover meant that it
became more appropriate to run from predators, so that longer
legs were more useful. Food was now mainly at ground level, so a
longer neck gradually evolved, to enable convenient grazing whilst
standing. Feeding while standing is an important aspect of predator
evasion for herbivores, as is a wide angle of vision. The toes
gradually disappeared, forming into a single hoof, which enabled a
greater turn of speed and was also useful as a defensive weapon.

Sensitivity probably also developed at this stage, as the flight
response from predators had to be instantaneous. This response is
still very prevalent in the modern horse, despite the fact that there
are few predators in Britain today that should worry a horse. Most
riders have experienced the 'knee jerk' lightning reaction to harmless objects, or perceived threats.

The other notable development was in response to the gradual
change of diet. The horse's mouth, dentition and digestive system

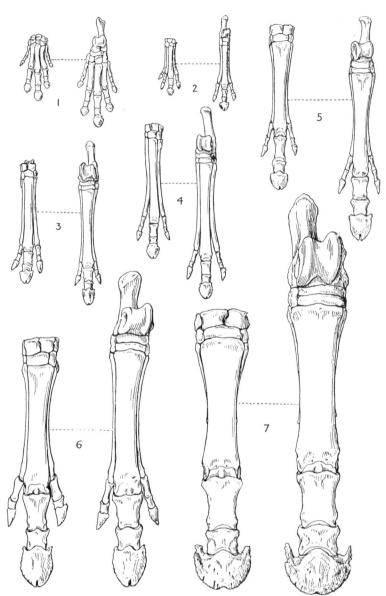

Comparison of the fore and hind feet of the horse with those of some of his ancestors numbered in chronological order. 1. Phenacodus 2. Protorohippus (Eohippus) 3. Mesohippus 4. Miohippus and Anchitherium 5. Protohippus 6. Hipparion 7. Horse.

The larger third digit has become increasingly dominant, whereas the rest have declined in both size and function. The earliest direct ancestor of the horse, Eohippus (c. 55 million years ago), is represented in Protorohippus, which had four toes on the forefeet, and three on the hind feet.

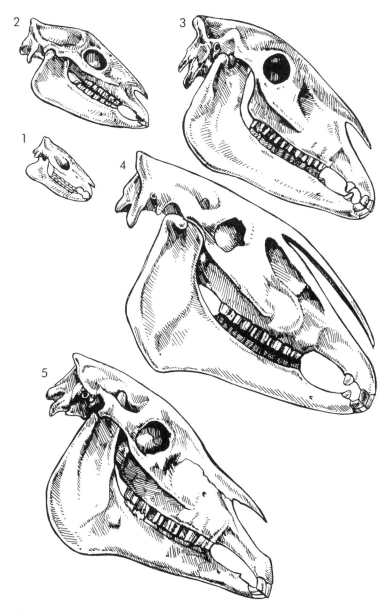

Skulls of the horse and his ancestors: 1. Protorohippus venticolus 2. Mesohippus Bairdi 3. Hipparion gracilis 4. Onohippidium Munizi 5. Arab horse.

The earliest of these skulls, which are in chronological order, dates back more than 55 million years, pre-dating mankind by about 50 million years. The huge jaw and tooth structure, which reflects the animal's reliance on high quantities of fibrous herbage, has hardly changed.

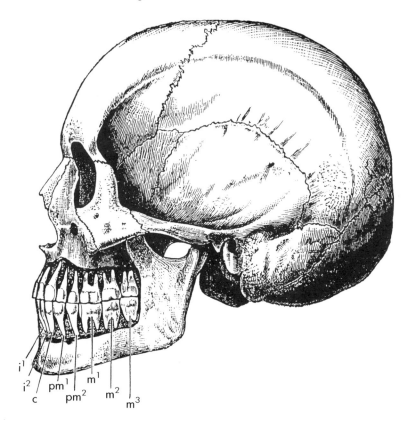

i^1 and i^2, incisor teeth; *c*, canine; pm^1 and pm^2, premolar teeth; m^1 m^2 m^3, the three molar teeth.

began to develop in order to make the best use of a low energy, high fibre, diet of varied but comparatively sparse herbage. The fleshy, whiskered lips and mouth became further developed to locate and identify specific types of herbage. The front teeth, or incisors, developed to slice off food to be transferred to the powerful molars for grinding. The teeth of the horse are open rooted, which means that they continue to grow in order to counteract the wearing effects of constantly grinding abrasive food.

The digestive process evolved for trickle feeding. This is common in herd animals of the plains, where food may be sparse. Such developments also help to preserve the flight response to predators. Large meals are not conducive to alertness and a good turn of speed.

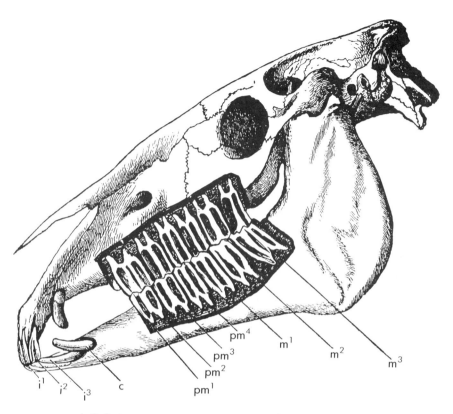

i^1 i^2 i^3, three incisor teeth; c, canine; pm^1, the situation of the first rudimentary premolar, which has been lost in the lower, but which is present in the upper jaw; pm^2 pm^3 pm^4, the three fully developed premolar teeth; m^1 m^2 m^3, the three true molar teeth.

(Left and above) The skulls of man and horse (showing complete teeth). The differences between the skulls reflect the diet. The horse's food is sliced off by the incisors, and then ground using the powerful molars. The horse spends a great deal of his time eating and the position of the eye means that he can watch out for predators while grazing. Man has a comparatively smaller jaw with a different arrangement of teeth, indicating a diet which requires less mastication. His eyes are close together and forward facing, a reflection of his early development as a hunter-gatherer. Note also the different sizes of the cranium.

Horses are commonly regarded as grazing animals, probably a reflection of the type of food to which they are mostly given access: grass. In fact they are more appropriately described as foraging animals, and they must receive a variety of herbage if they are to be fed in accordance with their evolved requirements.

As he has with most domesticated animals, man has taken the basic natural characteristics of the horse and adapted them for his own needs. The wild horse was a sturdy, athletic and intelligent animal which could be put to a number of physical tasks to ease the work burden of man. Through careful, kind and sympathetic treatment he became one of the most important animal companions to man. The ubiquitous horse-power was born.

The natural requirements of the horse must always be viewed against the many pressures that are exerted on him in the process of domestication. While the central issues here are nutrition and medicine, it is relevant to take into account the many other factors which have a bearing on the subject of holistic management. The following are areas where the evolutionary factors are of particular relevance and are often overlooked, or at least are not kept in their proper perspective.

Locomotion

The wild horse is a foraging animal constantly alert and with hair-trigger responses to avoid predators. He is always on the move in the wild, roaming the plains in search of a variety of food, and interacting with other members of the herd in play and fight rituals. He has periods of rapid movement and periods of grazing. He is even able to sleep on the hoof, owing to an adaptation of limb anatomy to support his weight while he is dozing.

In the domestic situation we confine the horse to a small paddock or stable, allowing regular periods of exercise or work, interspersed with long periods of more or less total inactivity. We protect his hooves with metal shoes, which rely upon human skills to be accurately applied or else cause damage to the foot. The capacity for the natural shaping of the hoof by wear and tear under normal activity patterns is lost. The art of correct shoeing is vital to healthy feet, limbs, and the whole physiology of the horse: 'no foot – no horse'. In order to harness the horse's work capability, we apply various forms of equipment: collars, saddles, bridles, and so on, which are bound to affect his way of going. The design and fit of such equipment is of paramount importance to health, well-being and locomotor efficiency.

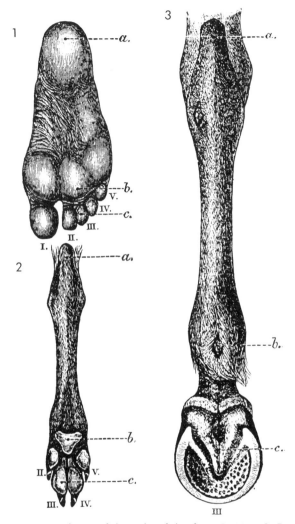

The plantar surfaces of the sole of the foot: 1. Man 2. Dog 3. Horse.
The illustration shows the 'sole' of the foot in each species, demonstrating
how anatomically similar structures have become adapted during evolution. This may be appreciated by comparing the various points, which
are represented in each case by the same letters and numbers.

In addition, of course, the riding horse has to carry a burden of
weight on his back and often perform feats requiring huge effort
and athleticism. Only good balance, understanding, and the skill of
the rider will keep the inherent risks to the health and well-being
of the horse at an acceptable level.

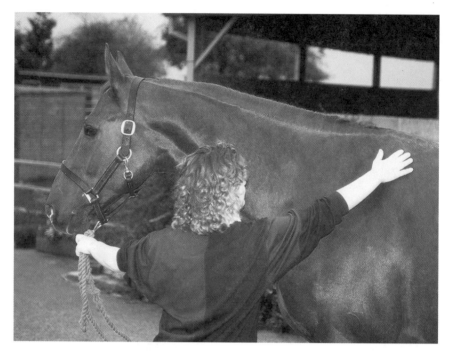

Imitating the horse's social behaviour increases our bonding with him. Scratching the withers signifies friendship.

Behaviour

By domestication we impinge on the horse's natural behaviour patterns. The herd interaction is prevented by single housing and single working. Horses paying attention to each other is not conducive to heeding human instruction, or the production of useful work. Horses' 'exercise routines' in a herd situation on the plains are not safe in the confines of a field or in close proximity to humans.

Dominance struggles are not viewed sympathetically, especially when one's own perhaps more submissive individual is injured by another horse putting it in its place. However, we tend to ignore the interactions that create a general sense of well-being, such as mutual grooming, formal and informal greetings, respect for 'space' and so on. These social niceties of the horse world should guide us in our approach to the handling of horses.

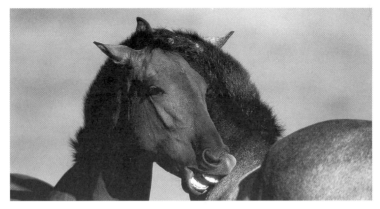

Mutual grooming is an integral part of the horse's social activities. By domestication we control these and other activities, denying the horse normal behaviour patterns.

Traditional feeding stuffs

Before the beginning of the twentieth century, the well-cared-for, sympathetically managed horse was arguably healthier and fitter than it is today. This is due to a number of factors, but nutrition is probably the largest single consideration. So many changes have taken place in British agriculture that our pastures bear little or no relation to those that used to exist. The horse often lives to a greater age than it once did, but this is probably a reflection of the fact that it is now kept as a companion animal without a purely financial value, rather than for commercial work.

The main differences between the diets of horses then and now are:

1. In modern pastures there is only a fraction of the species of grasses and herbage formerly found in most pastures.
2. No artificial fertilisers, pesticides or weedkillers would have been used on pastures or grain crops.
3. The horse would not have been fed compounded foods which have been denatured by processing and which contain artificial vitamins, sugars and other by-products.

The biggest difference in nutrition is certainly the variety of grasses and other herbage which used to be available to the horse. The vital nutritional contribution from multi-species swards and field margins are absent from most modern pastures. This affects the general health and well-being of the horse.

The application of artificial fertilisers has had the biggest influence on the number of herbage species. In one study conducted from 1967 to 1975 in Wiltshire, the average number of plants per square metre dropped by 36 per cent, from thirty-three to twenty-one – a loss of twelve species in just eight years (Nature Conservancy Council 1976). Farmers today apply nitrogenous fertilisers to grassland at twenty times the pre-war rate. Not only has this drastically reduced the species of flora, but in certain parts of the country the levels of nitrogen wash-off are becoming hazardous to health.

It is difficult to imagine what the countryside was like before modern farming methods changed it forever, but the works of John Clare written 150 years ago give a good insight. In Clare's day, most crops found their way back on to the fields as droppings or cattle bedding. Nutrients introduced in this way release their goodness slowly and in keeping with the natural order, whereas modern fertilisers encourage the rapid growth of certain species, which then smother others. They also cause displacement of important trace minerals from the soil.

Most pastures had rich hedgerows and margins, and often included some woodland, supporting many species of herbs and other flora. We know the varieties of pasture herbage which can be eaten by the horse *ad libitum*. Those growing elsewhere, which may have a more potent effect on the body, should not be given without qualified advice.

Our disregard of basic nutritional principles affects not only the health of the horse, but also many related areas including our own health via our food. It is only comparatively recently that we have begun to see the unfavourable effects of a 'chemistry set' approach to farming crops and feeding animals.

Until the 1940s, when horses were an important part of the commercial running of the land, their health and fitness was of paramount importance. Horsemen who knew their craft were highly regarded and comparatively well rewarded for their skills. However, not all their methods were humane by modern standards – in fact some practices were barbaric. Some of the methods used for minor veterinary problems varied from useless to positively dangerous. Remedies for worms, for instance, were often poisons of one sort or another, administered with little or no knowledge of chemistry or biochemistry. It seems likely that many horses were made ill as a result of these practices.

What these horsemen did understand, however, and put to good effect, was feeding. The relationship between diet, behaviour, and stamina was well understood. They also knew in general terms the effect that certain foods had on the physiology of the body (*The Farmer's Magazine*). Many formulae for compound feeds existed, designed for use under certain circumstances. Apart from the basic raw materials such as grains, locust beans and linseed cake, there were perhaps up to twenty other ingredients added. Many of them would come under the general description of herbs, although other ingredients such as antimony and sulphur were also included. These ingredients were all added for their therapeutic value. Some of the more exotic ones are not readily available today, and even if they were, expert knowledge would be required to feed them safely.

One of the advantages of feeding stuffs up to the 1940s was the provision of raw materials that were entirely 'organic', i.e. not subjected to modern chemicals, and therefore more wholesome than most of those available today. Pastures for grazing were a rich source of holistic nutrients. The benefits of putting a horse out in well-managed chemical-free pastureland meant that it was at liberty to browse on what it liked. Horses that were below par were often turned out to recuperate. Any dietary imbalance caused by the exclusive use of dried forage and hard feeds could be redressed in this way. Although the expression 'Doctor Green' is still used today, it must have had a real meaning in the past.

Apart from the benefits of the natural nourishment to be found in meadowland, other feeds were used in conjunction with hay to provide the extra energy for work. The best raw materials are those nearest to what the horse has evolved to eat, and horses would be in much better health if the quality of raw materials was higher today. We will now look at some of the feeding regimes and management practices at the beginning of the twentieth century and see what was fed, why, and how. Described below are the basic raw materials or 'straights' which formed the staple diet of many horses. As mentioned above, compound feeds were also used in a variety of circumstances. Most would have included other ingredients, such as ginger or turmeric and many others, or these may have been added as a supplement.

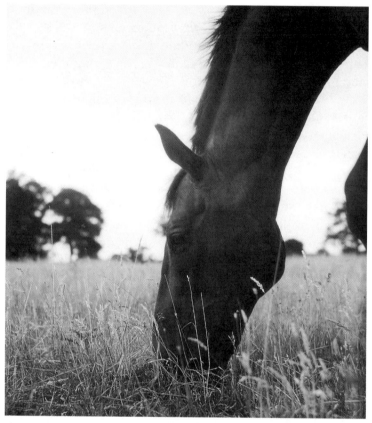

The position of the horse's eyes means that he has a good field of vision while grazing. This capability has evolved to increase his chances of evading predators in the wild.

Hay

As is common practice today, horses in hard work were limited in the amount of hay they received, although it was known that some hay should be provided to enable proper digestion. Chopped hay and straw (chaff) was often used to mix in with other feeds to slow down greedy feeders, and it was used extensively if the horse was fed from the nose bag during hours of long work. Hay was mostly chopped at home because, typically of the era, dealers were thought to be a thoroughly bad lot, often using inferior and damaged grasses.

The quality of hay depends on five factors.

1. The grasses and herbage of which it is composed.
2. The soil on which it has been grown.
3. The time at which the grass has been cut.
4. The hay-making process.
5. The conditions of storage.

Only the best hay was used for horses in fast work. It was moderately fine, hard, and sweet smelling, like new-mown grass. It would still be green and showing no signs of heating in the stack. It would be fed at no more than a year old and would probably contain flowers which still had colour, such as trefoil and clover, and many other species of herbage. The flowering heads of the many varieties of grasses would also be present, and the fibres of the best hay would lie in one direction if hand raked. The variety of grasses in the hay was directly related to the quality of the soil that it was grown on. This aspect was very important to horsemen who knew the value of having a good variety of herbage.

Lowland hay and water-meadow hay were not highly regarded if they contained neither the right species of grasses nor the rich variety of herbage.

Oats and other high energy ingredients

The amount of oats and other higher energy feeds was regulated according to the amount of work the horse was being asked to do. Oats are easily digested by the horse and because of this have been associated with heating or behavioural problems, although this is not necessarily so. They were regularly fed whole to mature horses, but they were also used crushed or rolled. Oats often made up the total concentrate ration of the feed, but other ingredients were sometimes used, such as peas, beans, wheat, and barley.

Bran

The chief use for bran was as a mild laxative, given as a 'bran mash', perhaps once a week. This counteracted the possible cons-tipatory effects of larger proportions of hard feed in the diet of horses in hard work. The use of bran has largely fallen out of

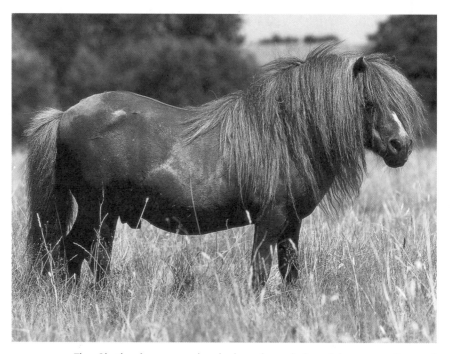

The Shetland pony, a hardy breed much loved by generations of children and adults alike. Full of character, though not known for an even temperament, they are still highly popular for riding and driving.

favour for a variety of reasons, but mainly because most people do not feed straights nowadays. Also modern bran is inferior to traditional bran and it has been linked to nutrient imbalances, but this arises from lack of basic understanding of balancing rations. Horses fed to a large extent on bran, unbalanced by other appropriate ingredients, can suffer many health problems.

Linseed

As with bran, the main use for this seed of the flax plant was as a mild laxative, but it could also be used as a conditioner. It requires thorough cooking before use to destroy potentially harmful enzymes, but contains useful protein and valuable oils.

These ingredients formed the staple diet of the horse, probably until the 1940s. There was nothing very complicated about the feeding of straights; it was only when materials such as therapeutic

herbs and other substances were used that it became more involved. The important rules were to use the best quality raw
materials, and to feed according to the work being performed, just
as is necessary today.

Myth, magic and a 'little something in the feed'

In addition to this basic diet, ingredients such as herbs and other
substances were used according to the desired result. In the days
before veterinary surgeons, the farrier was the principal horse
doctor and was charged with the responsibility of administering
medicines to the sick horse. The variety of treatments for various
ailments was endless, with the recipes for potions and powders
being handed down from father to son. Initially most of these
contained relatively simple ingredients, similar to those used in
human medicine of the time. As materials from other countries
became readily available, remedies became more exotic. The principles for their use were also influenced by foreign cultures, and
many strange and unfathomable substances were available to the
'horse doctor'. Some of these were useful, containing ingredients
which are the basis for some modern veterinary medicines; many
were valuable traditional medicines. However, a great number
were useless or dangerous, formulated by 'quacks'.

Several additions to the diet were given regularly in the feed;
these were not seen as remedies as such, but somewhere in
between food and medicine. Such things as garlic, nettle, carrots,
and cider vinegar were given in quantities which were quite safe
and were probably beneficial to health. The horse would normally
eat these ingredients quite readily.

Other additions, however, which were designed to have a
medicinal effect, were not accepted quite so readily by the horse,
and it can be appreciated why if some of the recipes are studied.
These concoctions often had to be administered by mouth in a
'ball', which was a blob of butter or other glutinous material used
to stick the ingredients together. The ball was administered either
by hand, or with a balling iron to protect the hand. The horse's
tongue was pulled forward, giving access to the back of the mouth,

In order to administer medicines which the horse would not eat voluntarily, ingredients were mixed into a ball, some of which were the size of a pullet's egg. An early-nineteenth-century recipe for a purging (laxative) ball is as follows:

7 drachms	Barbados aloes
2 "	Castile soap
2 "	Jalap
2 "	Ginger
1 "	Sassafras

Beat the whole into a ball with syrup of buckthorne.

As science progressed horse balls became more sophisticated (and safer). Later ones were wrapped in paper or gelatine capsules. There were various methods of administration but the basic principle remained the same.

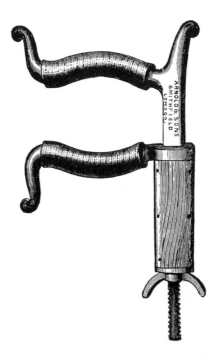

A horse gag, or balling iron, was used to hold the horse's mouth open during administration of the ball. They were not particularly effective due to the difficulty that the horse has in swallowing with his mouth open. However, they were used successfully during other procedures which also required the mouth to be kept open.

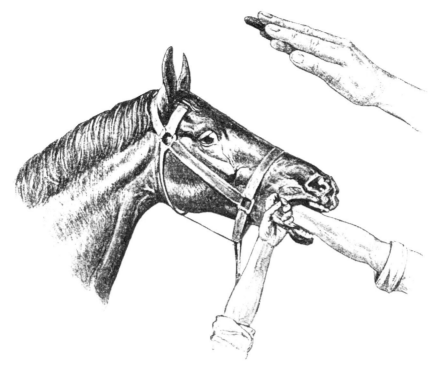

To administer a ball by hand, the ball is held by the right hand, while the left holds the horse's tongue.

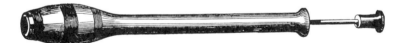

Balling guns worked on the simple principle of a child's pop gun. More sophisticated types had a spring and trigger mechanism. This one was used around 1900.

and the ball was placed as far back as possible, in order to get the horse to swallow it. Another means of administration, probably in use earlier, was a 'clog', which is a piece of wood put in the mouth like a bit, with honey or butter used to stick the ingredients on so the horse swallowed them gradually. Drenching was another option. This involved giving the medicines in a liquid form by mouth, holding the horse's head up during administration, so that he had little option but to swallow. Alternatively a stomach tube could be used to administer the medicines direct.

In common with human medicines, these potions could no doubt be traced back centuries. They were probably entwined with the supernatural or spiritual, as everyday life had a spiritual aspect that does not exist today in most western societies. An example of this is the 'frog bone' or 'toad bone' ritual, and although its origins are lost, it was still carried on both in Britain and abroad at least until the beginning of the twentieth century.

The ritual involved the use of a dead frog or toad which was hung in a blackthorn tree to dry. It was then buried to remove the flesh, and the bones were thrown into a stream. One of the bones of the skeleton is identical in shape to the frog in a horse's foot; and presumably because of its shape, it floated in a different fashion to the rest, and was thus identified as the magic hook or wishbone. The bone was crushed and mixed with various kinds of other materials, usually of a pungent odour. The resulting substance was then used for all manner of ailments, including the drawing of wounds. To the modern mind the story bears no relation to effective medicine, until we learn that the bones were mixed with some other ingredient, which may have been the 'effective' ingredient.

Francis Clater, pictured c. 1810, was apparently a conscientious and well-respected druggist, farrier and cattle doctor. He was also a prolific writer and his work gives us a valuable insight into the treatment of horses in his day. The following passage from *Every man his own farrier* reveals attitudes which are very different to our own.

'A Star in the forehead'
'An artificial star may be formed in a horse's forehead in the following manner: make two holes through the skin, two inches distant from each other, and two more holes at the same distance, straight across. The holes must be of such a size as will admit of an ivory or bone skewer being introduced into them: which must be worked about until the skin be properly divided from the horse's skull.'

Wire was then inserted through the holes to form a cross, and pitch was applied to the wound. This was then left in place for three days, after which the wires were removed and the wound allowed to heal.

There is hardly any reference to alleviation of pain during this procedure, or in Clater's description of other operations such as eye surgery. Where methods of restraint were deemed necessary the use of the twitch was recommended (see p. 104).

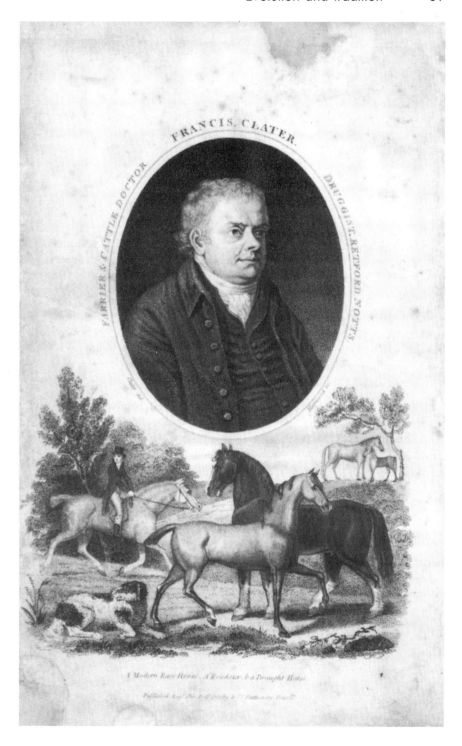

FARRIER & CATTLE DOCTOR   FRANCIS. CLATER.   DRUGGIST. RETFORD. NOTTS.

A Modern Race Horse, A Roadster, & a Draught Horse.

What the story also illustrates is a readiness to relate the power of positive healing to the horse. This approach, although ridiculed by modern science until comparatively recently, worked for man, so naturally he applied it to his horse. We now understand more about the importance of the mind in human medicine, but it used to be believed that the powers we now identify as important came from an external force, so they could also be invoked to heal the horse. There are many examples where the materials and methods used are explicable in modern scientific terms. For example, the fungal deposits from home-made preserves, such as jams, were used to encourage wounds to heal long before the discovery of penicillin.

Many traditional remedies had their roots in folk-lore and witch-craft, probably being modified by subsequent generations. Those which make some sense in the light of modern knowledge had a common theme of effective ingredients. It is a mistake to criticise out of hand everything which is not immediately explicable in terms of modern science. It is important to keep an open mind when making comparisons. What was done successfully may have been a result of luck, rather than of judgement, but it was none the less successful.

It is also a mistake to look to the past through rose-coloured glasses. Old-fashioned remedies often caused pain, misery and even death; there is no doubt that many horses were poisoned by the inexperienced, experimenting with toxic substances.

4

Nutrition and medicine

'Let food be thy medicine and medicine thy food.'
Hippocrates (c. 460−380 BC)

Principles and compromises

The holistic principle of nutrition and medicine is that they are in fact one and the same thing. This has been recognised since the time of the Greek physician Hippocrates, the Father of Medicine.

Food contains all the elements for health and well-being. As well as providing energy, certain foods have positive medicinal effects on the body, while others have negative effects. In order that optimum health through nutrition may be achieved, all raw materials used must be entirely compatible with, and relevant to, the evolved physiology of the horse.

'You are what you eat' is one of our most hackneyed expressions, and yet its true meaning is often overlooked. All creatures that exist on the earth consist of no more nor less than the natural elements of the earth. These are taken in as food by the body, or breathed in as air, as part of the process that has evolved for each particular species. The wholesome raw materials available from nature are entirely suitable for absorption and processing through the sophisticated chemistry of the body.

The body instinctively rejects all substances which are incompatible with its physiology. This function is part of the immune system which maintains the integrity of each individual; it is vital to the survival of all living creatures. The mechanism is remarkably sophisticated and will reject all non-compatible substances. This includes foreign materials in foods.

There can be no good health without good nutrition. There is no doubt that poor nutrition may be associated, either directly or indirectly, with many diseases. The body has an in-built regulatory system, so that it can cope with short-term imbalances caused in nature by an irregular supply of nutrients.

There are two aspects here which are important. Problems will occur if there is a deficiency of the right type of food, and also if there is an excess of the wrong type. In some cases associated problems soon become apparent, but it can take years for others to develop.

In nature, horses usually have direct access to fresh foods of the type with which their physiology has evolved to cope. In these circumstances there is usually no question about the suitability of the diet, selected by the horse on the basis of palatability and instinct. There is no doubt that this is the best way to maintain health and vitality. However, the horse, in common with other domesticated animals, now receives a large part of its diet from manufactured food. In addition the horse's diet needs special consideration because work requires extra energy which is not available from the low energy diet it receives in the wild. This energy is usually provided in the form of grains which are less compatible with the horse's physiology. They need to be fed with care in order to avoid problems associated with digestion and behaviour.

The manufacture of compound feeds involves processes which can compromise the ideal circumstances which exist in nature: storage of raw materials, cooking, and the use of artificial ingredients. Denatured by-products from other food manufacturing processes are often used, some of which are unsuitable. When these factors are combined, the risk of nutritional imbalance is greatly increased. Responsible manufacturers are aware of the implications and make allowances to try to reduce the effect of these compromises, but the fact remains that there is a compromise.

Apart from the compromises involved in the types of foods fed to the modern horse, the other major influence is the way in which they are fed. Horses have evolved as trickle feeders, as can be seen by watching them in pasture, where they spend most of their time with their heads down grazing. The stomach is relatively small, and most of the goodness from the food is absorbed during its passage through the gut. It is here that the bacterial population breaks down the material to provide nutrients for absorption by the horse. For this reason the horse should be fed little and often, which is not always practical for the modern horse owner.

When compared to its wild ancestor, or indeed to its modern wild counterpart, the domestic horse is probably as far removed from its natural environment as any other domesticated species. In the wild this highly strung, sensitive and intelligent animal spends most of its life browsing vast tracts of open country, through which it is free to gallop. The domesticated horse is usually confined in a relatively small field, and possibly stabled. In addition the components of his diet are far from his natural requirements. He often has to carry a burden of weight on his back, and sometimes jump with this load. Considering all this, plus the fragmented modern approach to many management issues such as nutrition and medicine, there is little wonder that the modern horse suffers from an increasing number of physical and mental problems.

Modern feeding stuffs

Many compound horse feeds and feed supplements contain raw materials which are less than ideal. Some contain ingredients which should never be used; products of animal or fish processing, for example. The responsible manufacturers do not use the worst of such ingredients, but some do, and when questioned can be very secretive about their products. A great many quasi-suitable ingredients may be used by manufacturers in formulating a ration in order to arrive at a final chemical analysis, ingredients depending upon current prices on world markets.

Because of the deficiencies in the diet of the modern horse, there are an increasing number of feeds and feed supplements available which claim to contain raw materials which will balance the diet. Many of these contain herbs, some of which should not be used on a routine basis. The majority of these products are not formulated on a scientific basis, and many do not declare the exact nature of their ingredients. The horse-owner has a right to know what is contained in all products being fed, but it is not easy to obtain the information.

The consumer is advised to use only those products which list the exact nature and quantity of all the ingredients, or one which has been granted a product licence under the Medicines Act or is a

Licensed Holistic Product under the BAHNM regulations (see pp. 68–9). Read the label, and if this does not contain enough information about the raw materials, a telephone call to the manufacturer may help. Demand satisfaction, and if there are any issues that remain unclear, seek an alternative product. This may seem a somewhat cynical view, but manufacturers are in business to sell their products, and they are expert at being 'economical with the truth'.

The information below covers a number of issues which are relevant to the manufacture and marketing of equine feeding stuffs and feed supplements. It is designed to be a guide for those wishing to evaluate the suitability of such products.*

Legislation

The majority of statutory legislation concerning the manufacture of equine feeding stuffs and feed additives is contained in a number of Acts, which are constantly being updated and amended. The main Acts are the Feeding Stuffs Regulations, the Medicines Acts, and the Trade Descriptions Acts. Naturally each piece of legislation is lengthy and complex. An understanding of their interrelationship is needed in order to apply even general principles to a particular product.

The Feeding Stuffs Regulations

The nature of the legislation
The Feeding Stuffs Regulations 1991, with subsequent amendments, is a Statutory Instrument of the Government. It sets out regulations which must be followed by manufacturers of all animal feeding stuffs. The regulations are under constant review by the Ministry of Agriculture, Fisheries and Foods, and there are some eighty pages of regulations arranged in various schedules.

The purpose of the legislation
There are various reasons for having such regulations. Public

---

* More detailed information on feeding stuffs and supplements, including raw materials and associated subjects, is available from the BAHNM. Licensed Holistic Feeding Stuffs and Supplements can be recognised by a symbol which is carried on all packaging.

health and safety are high on the agenda, as is animal health and welfare. There are also a number of regulations concerned with the disclosure of information which is considered to be of interest to the consumer. The Government consults the various manufacturing trade associations, as well as other advisers, when legislation is under review, as it does in other spheres. Amendments to the legislation are made to answer specific problems; for example, the use of certain meat by-products was banned from cattle feed as a result of outbreaks of the disease BSE.

The 'statutory statement'
This part of the legislation sets out how certain information, thought to be of interest to the consumer, shall be given. The information relevant to horse feeds is as follows.

1. The statutory statement must be displayed on every product. It must include specified information, set out and expressed in the required form, and it must be clearly separate from other information carried on the product.
2. There are two classes of information, one compulsory, and the other voluntary. Most manufacturers only declare the compulsory information.
3. The compulsory information, as listed below, covers the main points as they relate to most compounded equine feeding stuffs. Under more unusual circumstances, other information should appear, which has not been listed here for the sake of brevity.
a. The name and address of the manufacturer of the product.
b. Quantity.
c. Storage life.
d. Ingredients – expressed by name in descending order of quantity, or by defined generic description, e.g. 'cereal grains'.
c. Artificial additives, i.e. vitamins and other micro-nutrients, expressed as Internal Units (IU); also flavourings, preservatives and colours.
d. The description 'complementary feeding stuff' or 'complete feeding stuff', and instructions for use.
e. The species for which the food is intended.

Materials and their meanings

There are around 140 different materials listed in the Feeding Stuffs Regulations under the heading 'Materials and their meanings'. The majority of these are by-products of one sort or another. Most are drawn from other industries world-wide and many are routinely used in compounded horse feeds.

This area of the legislation gives rise to more confusion than any other. Many horse owners would not want to feed some of the raw materials used in certain compounded feeds, but sometimes their precise nature is not clear. This is because materials can be grouped by the manufacturer under a generic name; for example, the term 'oils and fats' actually covers 'oils and fats from animal or vegetable sources, and their derivatives'.

It is plain that some of the materials listed as by-products are more suitable for the horse to eat than others. 'Dried brewer's grains', for example, would probably be regarded as more suitable for the horse to eat than 'citrus pulp', which is all that is left of the fruit after the juice has been removed. It is also highly probable that many by-products from either fish or meat processing would be regarded by most people as unsuitable.

Responsible manufacturers will not try to conceal the type and source of raw materials used. Many are now reducing the amounts of some of the raw materials used in the light of medical and ethical considerations.

Sugars in horse feeds

The vast majority of compounded horse feeds contain sugars, mostly as molasses, or other by-products of the sugar refining industry. They are used as a cheap source of energy, they can disguise poor quality ingredients, and they can make inferior food more palatable. In some feeds the sugar content is as much as 10 per cent. Most people have got so used to highly molassed feeds that they accept them without question, perhaps thinking that because the smell and taste is attractive to the horse, it must be good for him. Some manufacturers try to justify the use of these materials by claiming that they are identical to the sugars found in the horse's natural diet. The vital difference is that added sugars are extracts, whereas any sugar should be part of the food itself.

Added sugars can alter the balance of the gut bacteria to a degree that may cause digestive problems and colic, immune imbalance and behavioural problems. If sugars are not added, digestion improves and the horse looks and feels better. For reasons best known to themselves many manufacturers do not like reducing sugars; however, there are now some feeds on the market which contain appropriate levels (see pp. 68–9).

The Medicines Act

Marketing authorisation

If a product intended for horses comes under the Medicines Act, it must have a marketing authorisation issued through the Veterinary Medicines Directorate. The product must satisfy strict conditions in the primary areas of quality, efficacy, and safety. These regulations are in force to control the manufacture and sale of such products. One of the purposes of the legislation is protection of consumers and the animals in their charge. Claims for the effectiveness of the product, and information carried on the packaging, are then strictly controlled by the licensing authority.

There have always been simple traditional feed supplements available, which have been sold for general use, rather than for a specific medicinal purpose. Such things as garlic and linseed oil, together with a host of other simple remedies, have been used for many years. These products are generally regarded as safe if used sensibly, or at least will do no harm to a horse in good health. They were never subject to the Medicines Act, because they were not sold for a 'medicinal purpose' in that the manufacturer made no claims for the physiological or medical effects of the product. The contents were perfectly clear, and there was no mention of any disease or condition. There is relatively little health risk in these circumstances.

The Trading Standards Department

The Trading Standards Department's duties are to improve and maintain standards of fair trading in terms of quality, quantity, safety and description. These duties are established by legislation laid down in Acts of Parliament.

The department carries out its duties through inspection, sampling, testing, and investigation. It will enforce legislation by prosecution if necessary.

It also informs, advises and educates manufacturers, traders and consumers. The department works closely with other government departments, as well as outside bodies.

The department offers free, impartial and strictly confidential advice upon enquiry, and there is never any reference made to the name of any individual making a complaint.

The Veterinary Surgeons Act 1966

The Veterinary Surgeons Act 1966 makes it illegal for any person who is not a veterinary surgeon to treat, or give advice for the treatment of, any condition or disease of a horse. There are no exceptions to this rule. Those qualified in allied professions, such as medical herbalists, nutritionists, dietitians, or nutritional therapists, must either work under the direct supervision of a veterinary surgeon or, if acting alone, must not treat or give advice for the treatment of any condition or disease. The Act is quite clear and unequivocal.

Practising veterinary surgeons will indicate their membership of their governing body, the Royal College of Veterinary Surgeons, by the letters MRCVS or FRCVS after their name.

There is an increasing number of therapists offering their services in various capacities. It is the responsibility of the owner of the animal to check on their qualifications. Owners seeking help from those who are not veterinary surgeons are liable to prosecution under Animal Welfare Legislation if allowing or seeking such help causes an increase in, or fails to delay, suffering and pain.

Holistic feeds

Holistic practices and principles in nutrition and medicine were defined according to the principles of the scientific theory of holism, first published by Jan Christian Smuts.

Equine feeding stuffs and supplements licensed by the British Association of Holistic Nutrition and Medicine (BAHNM) as holistic products can be identified by a symbol which is carried on all packaging.

The licensing scheme is administered through the BAHNM in collaboration with the Trading Standards Department and in consultation with others involved in legislation such as the Medicines Act and the Feeding Stuffs Regulations. The label acts as an assurance to the consumer that the product complies with 'Quality Standards for Holistic Equine Feeding Stuffs and Feed Additives'. They must be made according to strict protocols in order to ensure satisfactory standards in the primary areas of safety, quality, efficacy and nutritional viability.

The Association gives independent and impartial information through articles published in the equestrian press. It provides technical material and reference books, as well as a free telephone helpline for information on the following:

> Health issues raised by the use of inappropriate use of raw materials in feeding stuffs and supplements
> Consumer rights
> The Feeding Stuffs Regulations
> The BAHNM regulations
> Licensed Holistic Feeding Stuffs and Supplements
> The Medicines Act
> Licensed Medical Products
> The Veterinary Surgeons Act and the law concerning the treatment of animals.

Natural versus synthetic

Horses are foraging animals, a fact that is often overlooked. They are evolved to derive optimum nutrition from a wide variety of herbage as part of their diet.

If horses are fed naturally, nutrition is a relatively simple matter. However, the modern feed industry takes a different approach, which may involve compromises from a holistic point of view. The degree of compromise depends on factors such as raw materials, manufacturing methods, and storage. Each of these has an effect on the nutritional profile of the food, directly on the horse's intestinal micro-flora, and consequently on the mental and physical well-being of the horse.

In nature, animals normally consume only fresh foods. Domestication brings with it the necessity to store foods. While the general rule is 'the fresher the better', provided the feed is made from unadulterated raw materials and stored in good conditions food may be kept for a considerable time.

Our forefathers managed perfectly well in the middle of the winter feeding their horses on hay and hard feed from the previous year's crops. The practice of feeding horses in this way has fallen out of vogue, largely because it is not practical for the modern single-horse establishment. This fact, of course, creates a market for instant feed in a bag, where the responsibility for correct nutrition is taken over by the manufacturer. Food is processed, and this necessitates the addition of synthetic nutrients and artificial preservatives. Colourants and flavourings may be used to disguise unsuitable raw materials.

Manufactured vitamins and other micro-nutrients in modern compound feeds

It is important not to lose sight of the fact that it is entirely possible to manufacture feeds for all levels of work without using laboratory produced vitamins or other micro-nutrients, provided that the correct raw materials and manufacturing processes are used.

Supplementation of poor quality, or too few, raw materials with artificial products cannot reproduce the complex nutrient profile of holistic feeds. This is only possible through the use of un-adulterated raw materials, which should include specific species of herbage to provide quality sources of vitamins and other nutrients. Compound feeds formulated on these holistic principles (see p. 64) may contain around thirty raw materials; most others contain less than half that number.

Unfortunately, as we have seen, some modern horse feeds are manufactured from raw materials which, given the choice, horse owners would not set out to buy for themselves. They often contain raw materials which are alien to the horse's physiology, including high amounts of manufactured vitamins and other micro-nutrients in an attempt to revitalise the product. They may also contain up to 10 per cent sugar in the form of molasses. Such feeds are not prepared with due regard for what the horse has evolved to eat. Also the views of respected research establishments are often ignored.

The National Research Council, an independent scientific organisation, produces figures on the nutritional requirements of horses which are held in high esteem, or even as gospel, by most equine

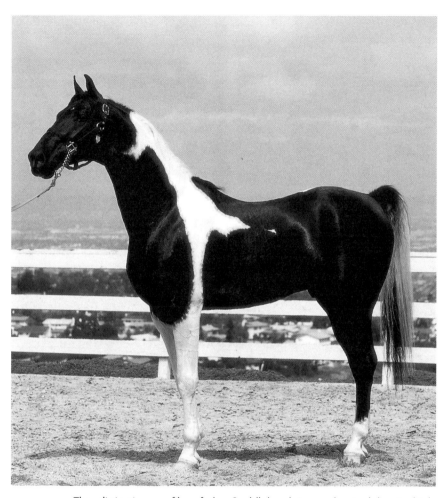

The distinctive profile of the Saddlebred is emphasised by its high stepping gait. It was developed as a breed in the United States and is a popular show horse.

nutritionists. They are prepared from a comprehensive pool of information from many sources world-wide. They are used regularly as a bench-mark for the manufacture of feeding stuffs for several species of farm and domestic animals. These data are informally known as 'the NRC figures'.

The NRC figures for horses begin by pointing out that many questions in equine physiology have not been solved (NRC, *Nutrient requirements of horses*, p. 1). A passage from the introduction reads: 'The sub-committee found large gaps in the published information, unresolved conflicting reports, and a disconcerting need to apply information gathered under one set of circumstances to very broad and diverse management systems.'

It recommends that horses should be treated as individuals. Many factors should be allowed for, such as digestive and metabolic differences between horses, health status, variations in the nutrient availability of the feed ingredients, and interrelationships of nutrients (p. 1). It goes on to say that the precise dietary requirements for (synthetic) vitamins A, D and E are not known (pp. 19−23).

Many recommendations for equine nutrition are extrapolated from work done on other species. The NRC recommends caution when making such assumptions: 'Some substances used in other livestock feeds are toxic to the horse. For example, monensin, which is an iodophore used as a growth promotor for cattle and poultry.'

Monensin can be lethal to horses when fed in amounts that would be safe to cattle and poultry (Matsuaka 'Evaluation of monensin toxicity'). Therefore any feed designed for use by other species should be evaluated carefully before being fed to horses (NRC, p. 38). Furthermore, extreme care must be exercised in milling, so that residues of previous foods containing monensin cannot reach horses.

The horse's physiology is entirely different from other agricultural species studied; and there have been no life-time studies on the cumulative effects of products currently being added to most compounded horse feeds. These reasons alone should exclude their use on a routine basis. It is a no-risk alternative to use raw materials which do not need fortification.

Vitamins

Vitamins are fragile yet potent chemical compounds. Together with many other elements present in tiny amounts they are known as micro-nutrients. When they are present as an integral part of raw materials used in foods, they may be termed holistic. When they are added from an external source which is largely out of context with the evolved requirements of the species, they may be termed non-holistic.

Vitamins are available naturally to the body, either in food or manufactured by the body itself from other food. Very little is known about some of the vitamins that have been isolated, and there are probably many more to be identified. So apart from the vitamins that we know most about, such as A, B Complex, D, and E, there are a host of others about which we know little or nothing.

They do not in themselves provide energy, but regulate a complex metabolism, through which other biological functions are carried out. The name vitamin was first used by a Polish chemist in 1911, derived from 'vital to life'. Although the presence of vitamins was known many years before then, their importance was emphasised with the rise of the modern food industry.

As science developed, it became possible to manufacture vitamins and other micro-nutrients, which could be used to 'fortify' denatured raw materials. Manufacture of vitamins and other micro-nutrients is a very sophisticated process. There are a number of manufacturing techniques employed, some of which use relatively simple methods, others which involve complex chemical manipulation, biological or genetic engineering and animal experimentation.

Their purpose

Vitamins are all so different from each other that a common description is difficult. They may be conveniently separated into two groups, water soluble and fat soluble.

They are important in many chemical reactions which play a part in maintaining good health. They enable complex chemical processes to start, and they have been shown to be associated with particular functions, such as reproduction.

Requirements

If the body is provided with food of the right type and quality, vitamins, as well as other micro-nutrients, are taken in as an integral part of the food. Each nutrient should be seen as part of a complex biological entity or 'whole', rather than in isolation. Food is more than just the sum of the parts.

The multiple interaction of these essential substances is the basis of their biological function, the adequacy of that function depending on the substances being supplied in the right mixture and concentrations. It is the relationship between the nutrients that determines their capacity for absorption and utilisation by the body, rather than the level of individual elements (Colgan, *Your personal vitamin profile*).

There are many aspects of biology which are not understood; nature contains factors which are vital to life, which cannot necessarily be reproduced in a laboratory. These two examples quoted by Sharon in *Complete nutrition* (p. 98) illustrate the point. The first is that salt-water fish will not survive in artificial seawater, despite the fact that it is chemically identical to real seawater. Secondly, in a human study, a group of patients suffering from digestive disorders were given extra B complex vitamins from a natural source. Their distressing symptoms were alleviated or completely cured. However, when the natural vitamins were replaced with laboratory-produced ones, the symptoms returned.

Manufactured vitamins

The sophisticated techniques of modern science mean that it is possible to supplement feeds with compounds which are chemically identical to natural elements. However, it is thought that the body still recognises these as foreign substances, and desired benefits have to be carefully considered against the possible side effects.

If artificial vitamins and other micro-nutrients are added to feeding stuffs, it is a legal requirement to declare the fact. This must be done within the Statutory Statement along with the other information as required by the Feeding Stuffs Regulations. They are expressed as International Units, a unit of measure which indicates the level added.

Many contra-indications are known for the human use of man-made products introduced into the body. No fewer than sixty separate items are listed as 'vitamin cautions' by the eminent human food scientist Mindel (*The vitamin bible*, p. 218).

Physiological considerations

1. They may contribute to deficiencies by preventing natural vitamins from performing their beneficial functions (Karic, *Vitamins*, p. 62).
2. They are known to be poorly absorbed by the system and are biologically less active. Poorly utilised by the body (Mervyn, *Thorson's complete guide*, p. 262).

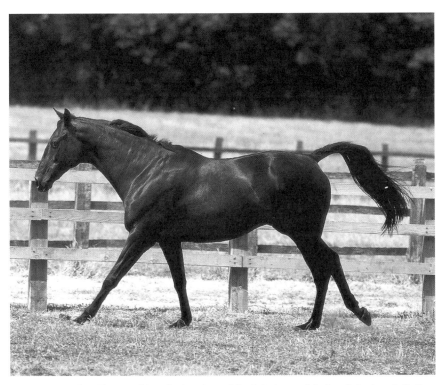

The Thoroughbred, developed in Britain and Ireland, is the definitive racing horse. It has been introduced into many other breeds intended for equine sports.

3. They are not retained efficiently in the body (Mervyn, p. 262).
4. They have no synergistic activity, which means they do not combine their activities with natural vitamins (Mervyn, p. 262; Sharon, *Complete nutrition*, p. 98).
5. Their effects on the body are not fully understood (Sharon, p. 98).
6. The addition of high quantities of specific and separate vitamins from an alien source probably upsets the overall nutrient balance (Mindel, *The vitamin bible*, p. 218). This can increase the risk of malnutrition or toxaemia.
7. They can compromise the immune system, as they may be recognised as foreign material.
8. They can cause toxic reactions (Mindel, p. 218).
9. No life-time studies have been done on equines, therefore the long-term effects are not known.

Natural vitamins

As we have seen, natural vitamins should be present as an integral part of the food. Like all nutrients, they have a complex synergistic interaction with other elements of the food, which synthetic products do not achieve. Such discrete relationships form part of the holistic nutritional profile, which must be maintained if the food is to be assimilated naturally and optimally into the body.

Benefits of holistic vitamins

1. They are better utilised than non-holistic vitamins, because they are taken in together with other nutrients (e.g. vitamin C and bioflavonoids occur in foods together, and function in the body together – Mervyn, p. 262). They also have a synergistic effect with other elements of the food (Mervyn, p. 262; Sharon, p. 98).
2. They are better absorbed by the system than non-holistic vitamins (Mervyn, p. 262; Ludwig, *Report on distillation product industry*), biologically compatible, and easily utilised.
3. They can be properly stored by the body for use later.
4. When part of a sensible balanced diet, they have no adverse effects on the body.
5. They are biologically more active than non-holistic vitamins (Mervyn, p. 262).
6. When part of a sensible balanced diet, they have no toxic effects.
7. They are retained by the body longer than non-holistic vitamins are (Mervyn, p. 262).

5

Holistic feeding

'A horse is what it eats.'

The basic principle of holistic feeding, as we have seen, is to feed raw materials which are as close as possible to what the horse has evolved to eat. For the horse-owner using 'straight' feeds, that is buying the individual raw materials for home mixing, it is a relatively simple matter. However, for the majority of owners this is not a practical proposition. Many people prefer to use compounded feeding stuffs, and the contents of most compound feeds are not easy to judge from a holistic viewpoint, as we have seen, other than with the help of the BAHNM licensing scheme.

What to feed

Horse owners who have the time, and can justify buying raw materials in economical quantities in order to avoid long storage, may wish to feed 'straights'.

Many owners will not use this method because of the risk of making a mistake, which may lead to nutritional imbalances or perhaps behavioural problems. However, a basic knowledge of 'straights' will help when making decisions about the purchase of compounded feeds and feed additives. Feeding 'straights' also has the advantage that the owner can find out by trial and error what suits a particular animal.

The only problem with feeding straights is that getting materials which conform to any common standard can be time-consuming and troublesome. Most ingredients available will have been sprayed with agricultural chemicals, and straights which have been pre-cooked may have been denatured by this process. Also, without specialist knowledge the types of herbage required and their inclusion rate may be a problem. It may be necessary to find up to thirty or more raw materials to feed a balanced holistic diet. In any event, those embarking on this type of feeding regime will learn a lot by asking questions about the various aspects of the straights that they are interested in.

The thing to remember with feeding straights is to keep it simple. Try to buy the best quality forage and concentrates, which conform to holistic principles if possible: no sugars – no synthetic materials – no crop sprays. Horses benefit from multi-species herbage, and if your pasture has been oversown with a few additional herb species, and has not been treated with chemicals, the nutritional quality will have been improved. However, as we have said, it will not be easy to 'turn the clock back'. Take qualified advice if you wish to supplement feeds with dried herbs, or fresh if you can get them. Always make sure that you know exactly what you are feeding, and why. In general terms there is no need to give any other supplements if diets are formulated to these principles. In fact the wrong type of supplement may well unbalance the ration. Many supplements, such as vitamins, are used at an alarming rate, and in some cases at levels which are toxic. Supplementation is not normally required if the horse receives the correct diet.

Feeds fall into two basic categories, roughage and energy food, or concentrates. The horse is designed to eat roughage only, but he requires energy food to support work. The energy food is usually given in the form of cereal grains or other materials which the horse's system has not evolved to cope with, and therefore they must be fed with care.

Traditionally horses were fed a diet of grass and hay containing multi-species herbage, together with oats and bran; the amount of oats was varied according to the amount of work being performed. As we have seen, the production of these ingredients is different now, and horses fed on them today may have nutritional imbalances.

The number of raw materials available for horse food today make the choice a bewildering one. It is important to make sure they are compatible with the horse's physiology, and many which are used in compound feeds are incompatible. The raw materials may have changed but the horse has not, and the basic principles

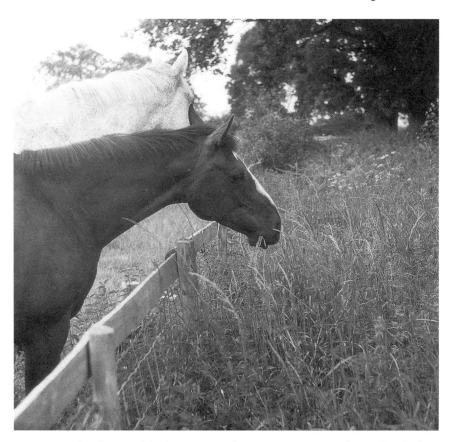

Depletion of herbage in modern pastures means that unless holistic rations are being given, many horses may be deficient in holistic nutrients. Signs of this are digging the ground, eating soil or tree bark, or simply picking at hedgerows for something they like. Problems usually only begin to develop if there is an imbalance or deficiency over a period of time.

of feeding remain the same:

1. Choose feeding stuffs which suit the evolved needs of the horse.
2. Feed according to the work level being performed, altering the ratio between concentrate feed and roughage accordingly.
3. Remember that the horse is designed to eat little and often; three feeds a day suit most horses and their owners.
4. Do not exercise immediately after feeding.

Holistic feeding takes account of the type and quality of all the raw materials, as well as the horse's physiology. The horse was not designed to ingest high levels of sugars, synthetic chemicals, or some of the by-products commonly used. Check that the information, which should appear by law on all packaging, is on the Statutory Statement. Sometimes the information is not expressed in a way that is easily understood, but most manufacturers are helpful. However, unscrupulous manufacturers, and indeed some reputable ones, may attempt to confuse or demean the enquirer; but the consumer has a right to demand and get satisfaction.

Roughage

The roughage element of the diet is the closest to the natural requirements of the horse, yet it is often neglected. A horse will thrive perfectly well on roughage alone, provided it is of the right type and quality. If the horse is not worked hard, concentrate feeds, that is grains, may not be needed at all. Traditional meadows provided all the nutrients a horse needs for good health, but most modern pastures are deficient in herbage species (see p. 50).

As an example, Table 1 demonstrates the number of species with pharmacologically active components in two types of grassland.

Table 1. Comparison of pharmacologically active components in two types of grassland

Compound	Traditional meadow	Modern pasture
Alkaloids	11	0
Glycosides	6	1
Essential oils	8	0
Tannins	8	1
Saponins	2	0
Pectins	1	0
Amara	3	0
Other specific	14	1
Phytoncides	10	1
Homoeopathic	39	0

One is a traditional meadow containing sixty species, and one is a typical modern pasture containing seven. The numbers represent the number of species which contained the relevant compounds. The table is simplistic in that the compounds are classified in main groups: there are many sub-groups, each member of which may demonstrate a different property. Alkaloids, for example, are a varying and diverse group, some of which are poisonous. It is obvious that modern pastures are deficient in many pharmacologically active substances. There is a close correlation between the profile of the diet and susceptibility to diseases; for the horse to maintain optimum nutrition and good health, the diet must contain all essential components.

Providing the horse with the varieties of herbage that are required for good health is one of the problems that the modern horse-owner faces. Lack of specific varieties of herbage which provide a comprehensive range of holistic vitamins, minerals and other micronutrients may have implications for health and the ability of the horse to maintain itself against disease. Pastures may be oversown with extra species (see below) which will go some way towards redressing the imbalance.

Dried herbal additives are also available. However, most of these are not formulated to appropriate specifications, their contents are often unknown, and their use can produce varying results, depending on the feed to which they are added.

The horse-feed industry responded to the need for added herbage by simply adding fragrant herbs, such as mint. Most of these feeds are described as herbal, but the manufacturer's rationale for adding herbs is largely to make the feed smell attractive, and to be seen to be catering for a return to 'natural products', rather than for any nutritional purpose.

There are a number of licensed holistic horse feeds and forage products available which redress the imbalances caused by lack of certain herbage and seasonal variations in feeding stuffs.*

Hay

Grass hay is usually divided into two types, meadow hay and seed hay. Meadow hay is cut from established pasture which may have been grazed at some time or other. It is usually softer and lower in

---

* Any feeds or additives claiming to contain therapeutic herbs should not be used unless they are licensed medicinal holistic products (see pp. 67–8).

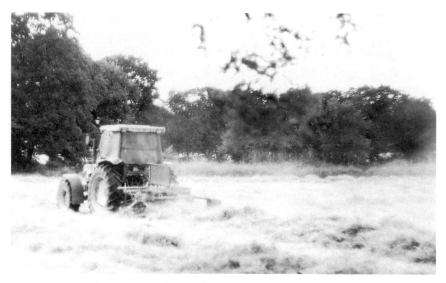

Modern hay is a far cry from that available before the 1950s. Current farming methods have reduced the nutritional quality due to the effects of land drainage and the use of modern fertilisers. Today it contains a fraction of the former species of herbage, which fact has many implications for the health of horses.

protein than seed hay. Seed hay is cut from meadows that have been specifically sown for hay making. It is of a rougher texture and higher in protein than meadow hay.

As in the past, the quality of hay depends on the types of herbage it contains, the soil it grows on, the time it is cut, and the conditions of making and storage. The main differences which affect the quality of the hay available then and now are: the lack of different species of herbage in modern pasture, and the fact that it grows on land which will probably have been treated with agricultural chemicals, which may poison and deplete it.

The quality of the hay is most important. It should smell sweet, and be free from dust when shaken, with no sign of mustiness. Fungal spores carried in dirty, poor quality hay can have serious implications when inhaled by the horse. Silage type feeds, that is semi-wilted grass conserved in sealed plastic bags, have evolved to try and solve the problem of moulds: these do not suit every horse, and digestive problems have been observed in some animals. There is no substitute for properly dried, best quality hay from traditional meadows.

Legume hay

Certain plants known as legumes have a higher level of protein than most types of grasses. Common types of legume are clover and sainfoin. The most popular legume for feeding to horses is alfalfa, also known as lucerne. It has been used as a horse feed for centuries in other countries, but has only recently gained popularity in the United Kingdom.

Lucerne is an excellent forage feed, which many horse-feed manufacturers include as a part of their compounded feeds. Most lucerne in this country is grown in East Anglia, and flash dried to maximise its nutritional content. Until recently the processing of lucerne included the use of relatively high quantities of molasses in order to keep the dust down, but some is now available with reduced, but still significant, amounts of molasses added.

Complementary herbage

We have seen (p. 80) that a typical modern pasture may be deficient in many vital elements and how this may be related to poor health. Floristically rich hay meadows and wood-pastures (woodland with areas of grazing) were the building blocks of Old English agriculture. Unfortunately there are precious few surviving primary meadows, the richest of which carry more than 100 species of plants. It is tempting to think that they can be re-created by re-planting and over-sowing existing grazing, but unfortunately it is not as easy as that. In order to appreciate why, it is useful to examine the underlying causes of the problem.

First let us define the word 'meadow'. Traditionally a meadow was grassland managed in a particular way to produce forage feed for the winter months. They remained ungrazed or 'laid up for hay' between the months of March and July. They contained not only the many species of grasses and herbage available in other pasture, but also those which flowered and set seed in early summer. They were usually sited on low lying land which was prone to flooding in the spring, and therefore not suitable for spring grazing, producing a rich crop later in the year. Meadows were regarded as being worth three or more times the value of other open land, and often covenants prevented them from being ploughed up.

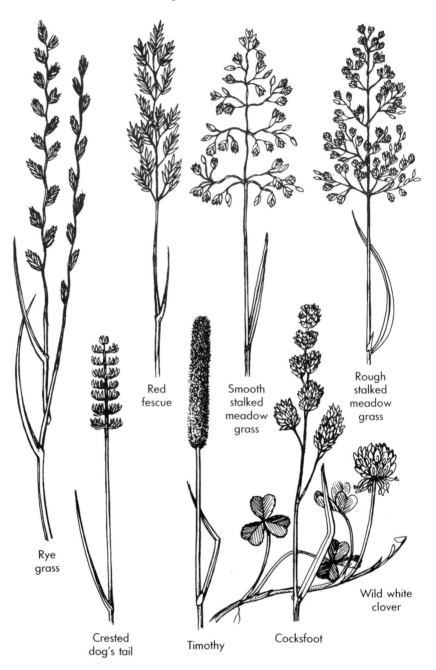

Rye
grass

Red
fescue

Smooth
stalked
meadow
grass

Rough
stalked
meadow
grass

Crested
dog's tail

Timothy

Cocksfoot

Wild white
clover

Grasses suitable for a horse paddock. Many other grass species plus a variety of specific herbage should form part of the horse's diet on a regular basis.

To put a field under the plough changes forever the basic structure of the soil, which has been relatively undisturbed since the field was created by clearing woodland ('field' is from Old English 'feld', meaning 'a felled area'). While the land can be re-planted it will never be the same again; it loses characteristics, developed over countless years, upon which many species of plants rely to survive.

In these days of order and conformity in farming we can only imagine the vast regional diversities in landscape which existed largely up to the second world war. The development of farming monoculture has changed the nature of the countryside completely – ploughing, fertilisers, pesticides, reduction of hedges and wild field margins, drainage of wet lands, and toxic waste have been the direct cause of the disappearance of floristically rich meadowland and wood-pastures. The knock-on effect of this is that many species of plants have disappeared (and with them many species of animals, birds and insects), which is the cause of the impoverished diet of modern grazing animals.

All this may sound rather gloomy but modern pastures can in fact be improved a great deal. Those taking the time and trouble to do so will gain many benefits, but it should be remembered that our efforts will be limited by the environment. We cannot easily re-create the grazing which took generations to evolve when the foundations of that creation have changed radically; we have to work with what we have got.

Many grasses and other beneficial herbage can be over-sown and will survive in existing pastures used as horse paddocks. The species used should not only be appropriate for the horse, but they should also be hardy and able to withstand grazing and cutting. They should have varying heading dates, which evens out the spread of growth, and the yields should not be so high as to upset the digestion. They should be of moderate fibre content.

A basic horse paddock mixture suitable for this purpose is:

Two perennial rye grasses (*Lolium perenne*): 50 per cent.
Two creeping red fescues (*Festuca rubra*): 25 per cent.
Crested dog's tail (*Cynosurus cristatus*): 10 per cent.
Rough or smooth stalked meadow grass (*Poa trivialis* or *Poa pratensis*): 10 per cent.
Wild white clover (*Trifolium repens*): 5 per cent.

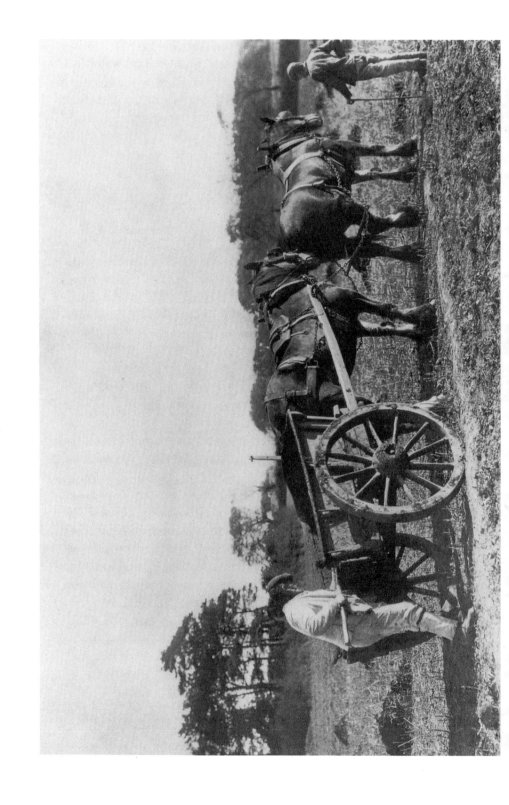

Other species, such as timothy or cocksfoot, may also be used.

Beneficial herbs which may also be included in this mixture are burnet, chamomile, chicory, daisy, dandelion, garlic, narrow-leaved plantain, nettle, parsley, vetch, and yarrow. There are many others which may be considered, and like those above their suitability will depend on a myriad of factors. The local ADAS (Food Farming Land and Leisure) office will be able to offer help and advice on local soil conditions and associated matters.

Once these species begin to get established, there are certain aspects of management which will assist in maintaining a desirable balance. Any overgrown plants, such as thistles and docks, can be thinned out if required. Total spraying of the field with weed-killer is not recommended. Manual removal is probably the best way but is not always practical; spot killing is effective, but should only be used as a last resort. As the balance between the species is gradually established the potential for one or two to become dominant at the expense of others will be reduced.

The use of artificial, inorganic fertilisers is not recommended because it causes certain species to grow faster than others, which then smother the slower growing varieties. However, some sort of fertiliser will be necessary at intervals, and soil analysis will help to decide how often this should be. Farmyard manure from cattle is ideal, but the type and rate of application will need to be considered in the light of local conditions (local ADAS will advise), and the pasture will need resting for some time after application. Horse droppings themselves are a fertiliser, but many owners remove them in order to reduce the worm burden. If they are harrowed, sunlight may have the same effect, but this is not always reliable. However, harrowing does go a small way towards fertilising the pasture.

Whilst the result may fall short of the grazing available during our forefather's day, pasture husbandry of this kind will provide much healthier grazing for the horse. Cultivating other species of herbage that the horse had access to in those days, particularly

(Opposite) When this picture was taken (around 1905), the droppings of farm animals were returned to the land as a valuable natural fertiliser. This practice declined as artificial fertilisers were developed, but its use was in keeping with the natural cycles of growth, preserving the rich variety of grasses and herbage.

those of wood-pasture, would be very unwise. Varieties which would have been found there, or the botanical equivalents, are probably best introduced as a supplement, which should be formulated by adequately qualified people. The therapeutic varieties should only be used for specific purposes as directed by a veterinarian. The proper nutritional or veterinary qualifications for formulating herbal supplements are rarely held by those involved in the manufacture of commonly available herbal products.

Poisonous plants
As a rule horses will not poison themselves with plants which contain toxins if there are other foods available, but there can be exceptions to this. The greatest risk is in weed-infested, horse-sick paddocks. The obvious sensible precautions are to prevent the horse from having access to poisonous plants, and to get rid of them wherever possible. The Ministry of Agriculture will give information on the poisonous plants that are likely to grow in specific areas of the country.

Toxicity of plants will vary according to several factors, such as the time of year, the soil conditions, and other food being eaten. Some poisons such as bracken and ragwort build up slowly and cause a gradual decline in health as the toxins accumulate; others such as yew can kill the horse almost immediately. While some species of toxic plants such as the foxglove can be used by physicians for therapeutic purposes, all the species listed below should be treated as potential poisons.

Poisonous plants which can be found in the United Kingdom are: alder, black bryony, black nightshade, bracken, buckthorn, celandine, columbines, cowbane, darnel, deadly night-shade, flax, foxglove, fritillary, greater corncockle, hellebores, hemp, henbane, herb paris, horsetails, irises, laburnum, larkspur, lily of the valley, lupins, meadow saffron, monk's-hood, pimpernels, poppies, potato, privet, ragwort, rhododendron, sandwort, soapwort, sowbread, St John's Wort, thornapple, white bryony, and yew.

The most common causes of poisoning are ragwort, yew, laburnum, and bracken. Problems which arise from the other species can be anything from a slight stomach upset to more severe problems. Hay should not be made from pasture infested with poisonous plants: wilting may cause an increase in palatability.

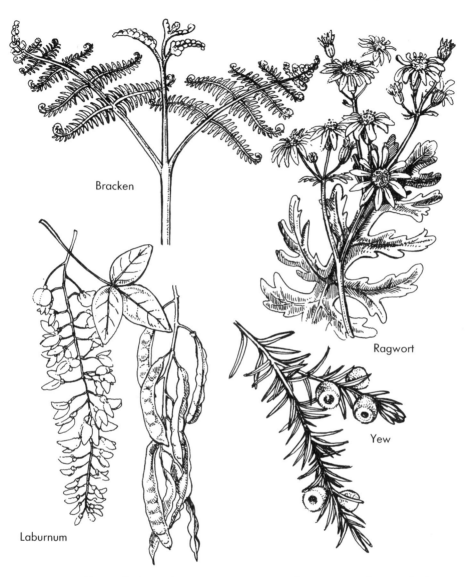

Bracken

Ragwort

Laburnum

Yew

Plants which are the commonest causes of poisoning in horses. A plant may poison directly, as a result of the chemical action of the tissues, or indirectly by impeding metabolism of vital substances. An example of indirect poisoning is bracken, which damages thiamine (Vitamin B1). Poisoning can also be a question of degree, depending on the severity of the toxicity. Sometimes the effect is so slight as to go unnoticed. It is thought that many horses suffer from the effects of mild toxicity possibly because they are forced to feed on poisonous plants in the absence of more suitable species.

Semi-wilted forage

This is grass that has been cut and compressed into plastic bags which are then heat sealed. The mild fermentation which goes on inside the bag effectively prevents any damaging fungal spores from developing. The result is an almost dust-free product, but in common with most agricultural crops, chemical products may well have been used on the product. These products do not suit all horses; a significant amount of diarrhoea has been observed in horses fed on them.

Straw

Horses with efficient digestion and good teeth may be given small quantities of wheat or barley straw; it is a good source of fibre. Because it has little nutrient value it should not be more than a very small proportion of the diet. Again, the problem with using straw is that it has probably been sprayed with agricultural chemicals.

Chaff

In former days the horse's concentrate ration was bulked up with 'chop' or chaff in order to stop the horse bolting the feed, and to encourage thorough chewing. The chaff was usually hay or straw. The modern equivalent is molassed chaff, which is available separately or already included in compounded rations. Molasses is added mainly to keep the dust levels down during manufacture; the use of molasses is now thought to be associated with digestive and other problems in some circumstances. While this is probably a matter of degree, there is no point taking the risk when it can be avoided. More products with less sugar, or even better no added sugar, are becoming available.

Concentrate feeds

Concentrate feeds, which are the part of the ration least compatible with the horse's physiology, must be fed to provide the extra energy required for work. They should be fed with care and consideration if digestive and associated problems are to be avoided.

Most grains can be fed whole, but if the horse does not have good teeth they will go through the system unaltered and unused. When manufacturing compound feeding stuffs it is common practice to clip, crush, bruise, cook, or a combination of these processes in order to make the nutrients more available to the digestive juices. Thus 'damage' to the grain creates the need for preservatives.

As soon as the grain is opened, it begins to lose its nutritional value, and cooking depletes it even further. Food compounders who cannot maintain the micro-nutrient viability from the raw materials used commonly add synthetic vitamins and other micro-nutrients. The presence of these may be confirmed on the Statutory Statement, their quantities being expressed as IU (International Units).

The traditional way of cooking grains for animal feeds is steaming, but the most commonly used method today is micronisation, or 'micro-waving'. Another method is extrusion, where the grain is cooked by impregnating it with steam and forcing it through dies to produce the familiar nugget shaped lumps. The high temperatures reached during this process destroy the majority of vitamins and other micro-nutrients, and feeds produced in this way are commonly fortified with synthetic products.

Oats

Oats are the traditional grain food for horses. They can be used as the total concentrate part of the feed, provided the diet as a whole contains the right amount of different herbage. They have been associated with heating problems, and must be fed with care in this respect, although this is not a consistent finding. They are best fed either rolled or crimped, although horses with good teeth can cope with them whole. The advantage of feeding them whole is that crimping or crushing can reduce their nutritional quality. Naked oats are a development of the ordinary variety which lose their hulls during harvest. They contain up to 27 per cent more energy than ordinary oats, weight for weight, and must be fed accordingly.

Barley

Barley is known as a fattening feed. It contains a higher starch level than oats and if fed uncooked it should be crimped so that the nutrients are available. Boiling is also a suitable method of preparing it. When supplied as part of a concentrate ration it is usually cooked by micronisation or sometimes by steam, and extruded barley is also available. These products may also contain synthetic vitamins, because the heat involved in the processing depletes the holistic ones. Some horses appear to have a reaction to barley and develop lumpy swellings or filled legs if it is fed to them. Like oats, barley can be fed to supply the total concentrate ration of the feed, provided the total diet contains the right amount of different herbage to balance and regulate this high energy feed.

Maize

Maize also has a reputation for being heating. Like other grains it may be fed whole to horses with sound teeth. When supplied as part of a compounded feed, it is normally steamed and rolled. It is a good conditioning feed and it can be used as a fair proportion of the concentrate ration.

Soya bean meal

Some raw materials are particularly useful for providing high levels of protein and soya is one of them. It must be fed cooked, and is pre-cooked if supplied as part of a compounded feed. Soya bean meal can contain up to 50 per cent protein. It can be used as the sole source of supplementary protein in the diet.

Linseed

Linseed is also used as a good source of protein, and it must be cooked before feeding. It is generally about half the protein content of soya. If included as part of a compounded feed it will be pre-cooked. Linseed can be used as a laxative and it is a good coat conditioner on account of the valuable oils it contains. While it contains about 20 per cent protein it should only be used in very small amounts.

Peas and beans

These are usually supplied pre-cooked by micronisation or perhaps steam. They contain about 30 per cent protein. They are commonly used in compounded feeds. They can be heating, and should only form a very small part of the concentrate ration.

Sugar beet

Sugar beet is normally supplied as dried pellets or shreds, which must be soaked before use. It is commonly fed to many types of horses, providing them with instant energy in the form of sugar, and also slow release energy from the fibrous content. It has an energy content similar to oats, and has the added advantage of being economical. Products containing added sugars are falling out of favour with holistic veterinarians, as they may be linked to digestive, immune, and behavioural problems.

Compounded feeds

This term covers coarse mixtures and cubed or pelleted products. The disadvantages of using cubed or pelleted products is that the quality of the feed is not obvious to the naked eye. Coarse mixes are increasingly popular with horse owners largely because they can see what they are giving their horse to eat. The disadvantage of coarse mixtures is the practice of including up to 10 per cent molasses or syrups, which many manufacturers do. In some cases, particularly during cold weather, the feed actually sets in the bag.

As we have seen the vast majority of compounded feeds, both coarse mixtures and cubes or pellets, contain synthetic vitamins and other micro-nutrients which are not in keeping with holistic nutrition. Apart from the nutritional aspects of these products, many horse-owners wish to disassociate themselves from the laboratory animal experiments involved in their production. In addition, some compound feeds may contain products which the horse-owner would not choose to buy for the horse, such as by-products.

By-products from a variety of sources are commonly used in horse feeds, included as a cheap source of raw materials. They are usually denatured and have to be chemically fortified. There is a huge number to choose from, and some of them are more compatible with horse physiology than others. Many of them, such as citrus pulp, would not be chosen by the horse-owner setting out to buy ingredients.

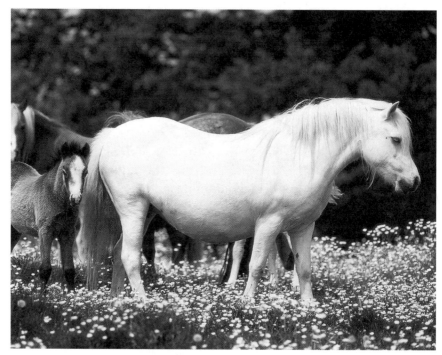

Welsh mountain ponies are a small but robust breed popular for children's ponies and showing; they stand under 12 hands high.

Although increasingly rarely, by-products from the animal and fish processing industries do find their way into horse foods and supplements. These are condemned by holistic practitioners, and probably by most horse-owners. Often the presence of by-products and also synthetic products goes undetected. Some information is available from the feed label on every bag, but it is not always very revealing, and specialist knowledge and information is required.

Molasses

Molasses is a sticky thick black liquid which is a by-product of the sugar industry. It will be found in many compounded feeds, forage products, and sugar beet. Other sugar products are also used under different names, such as syrup. Holistic veterinarians are recommending that such products are totally excluded from the horse's diet.

Water

Water must be taken into consideration as well as food. The quality of the local water supply will vary at different times of the year. As well as being hard or soft, natural water supplies can be contaminated from many sources, such as farm chemicals, sewage, industrial waste, or seepage from land-fill sites.

Tap water is a different matter, but it will still vary in chemical make-up depending on the time of the year and the area of the country from which it comes.

A constant supply of clean fresh water must always be available for the horse. Automatic drinkers are very useful and save a lot of time and effort, but as with buckets they must be kept clean. Plastic containers for holding water may not suit all horses.

How much to feed

The amount to feed a horse must be calculated according to the weight of the animal and the amount of work being performed. Feed companies are a good source of information for particular types of feeds, but remember they are in business to sell their product. It is probably better to consult an independent organisation or take advice from someone on personal recommendation. There

Table 2. Guide to approximate bodyweight

Height	Bodyweight in kg	(lb)
11 hands	120−260	(264−572)
12 hands	230−290	(506−638)
13 hands	290−350	(638−770)
14 hands	350−420	(770−924)
15 hands	420−520	(924−1144)
16 hands	500−600	(1100−1320)
17 hands	600−725	(1320−1595)

are a number of independent organisations which will give free
advice. Their names appear at the back of the book.

Generally a horse will eat about 2.5 per cent of his body weight
per day, calculated as dry matter; in other words the weight of the
moisture in the food must be subtracted. The figures are just a rule
of thumb. Some horses need much more, others do well on less.
Table 2 shows how to calculate the weight of the horse in order to
work out the daily dry matter ration.

*Table 3. Forage—concentrate ratio for different
work levels*

Work level	Hay (%)	Concentrates (%)
Resting	100	0
Light work	75	25
Medium work	60	40
Hard work	40	60
Fast work	30	70

Having calculated the total amount of feed required per day the
next step is to decide on the ratio between the roughage and the
concentrate. This will depend on the amount of work being performed, and can be calculated from Table 3. Thus a three-quarter-
bred horse, of about 16 hh and weighing around 500 kg, should be
fed according to Table 4.

*Table 4. Suggested feeding for a Thoroughbred-
type horse (16 hh, 500 kg)*

Work level	Hay kg	(lb)	Concentrates kg	(lb)
Resting	12.5	(28.0)	0	0
Light work	9.0	(21.0)	3.5	(7.0)
Medium work	7.5	(16.8)	5.0	(11.2)
Hard work	5.0	(11.2)	7.5	(16.8)
Fast work	3.75	(8.4)	8.75	(19.6)

6

Natural or alternative medical therapies

'Peruvian [Cinchona] bark, which is used as a remedy for intermittent fever, acts because it can produce symptoms similar to those of intermittent fever in healthy people.'

Samuel Hahnemann (1790)

As in human medicine there are a number of natural therapies available for horses. Some of these are accepted by the modern medical establishment, some are not. Although more natural therapies are now being recognised, it takes a considerable time to break down conceptual difficulties and the barriers of prejudice.

Some of these therapies have been established for thousands of years, but have only very recently been accepted by conventional Western medicine. For example, the Faculty of Homoeopathy at the University of London now trains veterinary surgeons in homoeopathy through a post-graduate course.

Another example is the acceptance of safety and therapeutic claims for magnetic therapy by the US medical licensing authority, the Food and Drug Administration, which is regarded as the most stringent body in the world. It is interesting to note that a theory of how the therapy works was formulated as a result of the American space programme.

Two of the most important aspects that separate many natural and traditional therapies from modern Western medicine are, first, the importance of treating the patient as a whole being, rather than treating the individual symptoms of disease, and secondly, the importance of incorporating symptoms of the mind in the healing process.

Western medicine does not generally accept principles which cannot be explained in its working medical language. Some of the practices that were previously classed as 'alternative' are now being understood in those terms and accepted. Often when presented with ideas which do not fit in with accepted science it is tempting to dismiss them. Modern science, however, should work alongside holistic practices and medicine so that both may benefit.

One of the main causes of confusion and condemnation of alternative therapies is unqualified practitioners setting themselves up as experts. Even leaving aside the legal aspects, the criticism is quite justified. There are many therapists claiming to use holistic methods involving the use of potentially dangerous substances, and in some areas, such as herbal medicine, there are no qualification standards for equine therapy. The consumer should be aware of the Veterinary Surgeons Act which makes it illegal for any person who is not a veterinary surgeon to diagnose and treat any condition or disease, whether by modern drugs or traditional natural medicines.*

The holistic practitioner has many methods of treatment available, all of which are entirely compatible with and support the natural processes of the body. They are not invasive in the way that pharmaceutical products can be, and therefore do not give rise to side effects. They include acupuncture, homoeopathy, herbal medicine, manipulative therapy, radionics and, of course, nutritional therapy, which may include the use of herbs.

The knowledgeable owner will want to make use of some of these practices in everyday management and there are many ways of doing this, provided the owner knows the principles involved. The use of herbs in feeding stuffs is a good example.

Herbs may be used in a variety of ways to help maintain good health. However, when they are being used as part of a medical therapy, the recommendations of a veterinary surgeon should be followed. If the owner wishes to follow holistic principles it is obviously best to contact a veterinarian who is practising holistic medicine.

The subject of alternative therapy covers a wide area of disciplines, many of which are overlapping. Listed below are some of the holistic therapies which are becoming increasingly available for horses.

---

* Guidance and advice on suitably qualified holistic practitioners may be obtained through the BAHNM.

Acupuncture

The basic theory of acupuncture stems from the oldest medical textbook known, the *Huang Ti Nei Jing Su Wen* or *Yellow Emperor's Classic of Internal Medicine*, whose precise age is unknown, but which is thought to date from several centuries BC. Chinese medicine treats the body as an 'energetic whole', rather than as a collection of separate components which present the physician with a specific disease. This whole comprises integrated and balanced components which function in harmony with each other and the environment when in good health.

Disease is considered to be simply an imbalance in the body, causing a deviation from health and harmony. Successful treatment of disease depends upon the practitioner's ability to re-balance the body. The basic Chinese philosophy of life involves the vital balancing principles of Yin and Yang. In medicine this is related to Qi, or what is known in Western cultures as 'energy'.

In health we consider the body's energy, or Qi, to be in balance in terms of Yang and Yin, the different polarities representing energy: positive−negative, hot−cold, dry−wet, male−female, light−dark etc. These fundamental components and the balance between them are used as a perspective to explain not only the workings of the body, human or animal, but also the way the earth functions, and even the universe.

Yin and Yang must be in correct balance for normal function. There is no absolute Yin and no absolute Yang; there is always Yang within Yin, and conversely Yin within Yang. Yang and Yin co-exist and flow from one to the other, but neither causes the other. This simplistic explanation of the natural order of things is far removed from the Western way of thinking. The application of some of the concepts can be difficult for Western minds to grasp, let alone accept.

The Qi, composed of Yin and Yang, flows through the body on a regular twenty-four hour cycle (circadian rhythm), channelled through what are called meridians. There are twelve main meridians on each side of the body, each related to a particular organ or organ system. If Yin and Yang become unbalanced, or the regularity of flow is disordered, then we have disease.

The mechanism of disease is also explained in simplistic terms. What are called 'pernicious influences' impinge on the body and its internal organs through the meridians. Such influences can be climatic, nutritional, emotional, traumatic or a variety of other factors.

The treatment of a disorder or imbalance is by correction of the Yin–Yang balance and the restoration of normal energy flow, or Qi. This is achieved by the use of herbs and nutrition, each strategy tailored to the body's need in terms of Yin and Yang, and by local stimulation techniques using fine needles, moxibustion (which involves heated needles), massage, laser, and electrical methods, all applied to specific points along the meridians. Correct treatment with lasting effects depends upon tailoring the techniques used to the needs of the animal. It is an essentially integrated approach requiring the support of nutrition and internal medicine. Acupuncture alone is not a complete system of medicine, therefore; traditional Chinese Medicine incorporates needling, nutrition, Chinese Herbs, and life-style philosophy.

The prime purpose is to stimulate the body's own healing powers, which are often underestimated by our modern society, and its ability to maintain its own equilibrium in its internal environment. The acupuncturist is far less concerned with the specific scientific name of the disease than with the nature and degree of imbalance. The predisposing and causative factors also need close attention to ensure good healing and greater permanency of cure.

All of this intricate understanding of the body and the well-proven methods of cure were worked out in ancient China by a tradition of close astute observation from outside the body. This is opposite to the modern methods of investigation which delve more often into the internal and microscopic changes in the body.

Internal symptoms are related to external pernicious influences, and consequent detectable changes in the meridians and acupuncture points on the outside surfaces of the body. Similarly, cure is effected through the same externally situated sites.

In addition to the twelve meridians on each side of the body, secondary meridians form interconnections while others spread in a fine network over the surface of the body forming the 'capillaries' of the system. These connections ensure an even distribution of Qi, and the balance between Yin and Yang: they also connect the internal organs to the body's surface so that Qi is carried from them to all parts of the body.

Diagrams of the meridians show them lying on the surface of the body, but in fact they lie at various depths, only coming to the surface in certain places.

Needles used for acupuncture are different from hypodermic needles used for injections in modern medicine. They are solid and rather finer in diameter. Because of this they are extremely flexible and can withstand any bending that occurs due to the action of the muscle tissue they are inserted into. Breakages are extremely rare. They are sterile to prevent the danger of infection and they are made in a variety of materials, diameters and lengths. Stainless steel is most common, but gold, silver and copper are also used depending on whether a stimulating or suppressing effect is desired. Needle lengths vary, because different acupuncture points are located at different depths in tissue; the shortest is half an inch, and the longest is twelve inches, although this is seldom required.

As well as stimulating the body's own healing powers and its ability to maintain its own inner balance, predisposing and causative factors also need to be investigated and eliminated to ensure good healing and to prevent recurrence. Before beginning treatment a good practitioner will spend time investigating the horse's history. In order to form an accurate picture of the problem and the best way of dealing with it, other factors must be taken into consideration besides the immediate clinical symptoms. These include the general physical and mental state, temperament, appetite preferences, work routines and environment. Advice will probably be given on diet, exercise, saddlery and shoeing, if it is felt that changes here will be of benefit.

Having decided on the most appropriate acupuncture points to use, the needles are inserted as quickly and painlessly as possible so as not to cause discomfort, which could adversely affect the patient's response and make it more difficult to treat. Provided the patient is fairly relaxed the insertion is relatively painless, with little more discomfort than that caused by a mild pin-prick. Very often, horses will accept the treatment very readily, or even enjoy it.

Acupuncture points vary in size, some being the size of a fifty pence piece, whilst others are just pin points, and are located by the practitioner noting differences in temperature, tension and tissue resistance. The most difficult points to find are those in the lower limbs or facial area. Exact points must be located if maximum effect and benefit are to be gained. Once the needles are in place, the points may be further stimulated by rotating each in turn, or by changing the depth by using an up and down movement, known as 'pecking' by the Chinese.

A resistance may be felt due to muscle grasp, which usually indicates that the correct point has been located; this may be surprisingly strong, making it very difficult to move the needle, but within a few minutes the grip will be released, making it easy to withdraw the needle again.

Other aids to the practice of needling are electro-therapy or moxibustion, where the herb moxa is wrapped around the needle while it is in position and ignited. The aroma from the herb plays an integral part in treatment, as does the warming effect of the needle.

Length of treatment may vary from five to thirty minutes, generally averaging fifteen to twenty. Horses rarely object to acupuncture; while a few may not be keen at first, most accept it well, progressively relaxing once the first few needles are in place. Cold laser can be used to stimulate acupuncture points with more fractious animals. Blood is rarely drawn, as care is taken to avoid blood vessels; hence the need for the practitioner to have a thorough knowledge of anatomy.

Most horses show signs of great relaxation during and after acupuncture, some even becoming drowsy. If the treatment is likely to prove successful, the horse will usually respond promptly, showing relief from pain or a lessening of symptoms fairly quickly. The response can be within a few minutes or it can be a few days. Initially the response to treatment may only last for a short period, but a favourable response to the first few sessions usually indicates that the animal is a good subject for such treatment and likely to benefit from further sessions, when the improvement should be of longer duration.

Sometimes a less favourable response is seen, with a worsening of the symptoms. While this seldom lasts for more than forty-eight hours, it usually indicates a hyper-sensitivity to acupuncture, and future treatments should be made shorter and carried out with care to achieve less stimulation.

Acupuncture is often perceived mainly as a method of alleviating pain but, when integrated properly with internal medicine and nutrition, it is perfectly capable of restoring health in the face of many serious and complex internal diseases. Locomotor and musculo-skeletal disorders are very suitable applications, and COPD, laminitis, colic, metabolic complaints, and skin diseases, among others, can all respond well.

Acupuncture is of course a residue-free treatment, so cannot contravene any rules of competition or racing. It is therefore becoming very popular, not only because of its justifiably burgeoning reputation for success, but also for its ability to help disease without any danger of breaking competition rules.

This popularity has its disadvantages, in that it can encourage a superfluous use of acupuncture techniques by those without a full appreciation of the subject. It is not yet widely used by the veterinary profession in the United Kingdom, and this fact encourages its illegal use by practitioners who are not veterinary surgeons. It must be remembered that if the maximum effects are to be obtained by following the philosophy and principles of this ancient practice, proper preventative management, nutrition, shoeing, and saddling must be practised; along with an appreciation of the fact that, although short-term relief may be gained, a longer term view is more beneficial.

Apart from the legal considerations it is in the best interests of the horse and the owner only to consult veterinary surgeons if this treatment is desired. They alone can carry proper insurance against mishaps, and keep an overview of the medical situation.

Happily, acupuncture, for centuries providing reliable first-choice medicine for a large proportion of the world's human population, is now much more readily available for horses, who have proved particularly responsive to and appreciative of its methods.

While not a universal remedy for all illnesses, a wide range of veterinary problems in horses can be treated using acupuncture, either on its own or in combination with herbal, homoeopathic, or chiropractic therapies. It should be remembered that the Chinese use acupuncture only as part of traditional medicine, not as a complete system in its own right. For this reason simply using needles alone may be insufficient for a good result.

Using more than one type of therapy can, however, sometimes cause conflict, especially if more than one veterinarian or practitioner is involved. To avoid this, when all the areas relevant to the problem are being considered by an holistic veterinarian it is important that those who have an input to make, such as the farrier or chiropracter, should work in consultation with each other. This should always be under the auspices of the veterinary surgeon so that the treatments and their effects can be correctly integrated, monitored and assessed. In this respect, it is often more convenient and effective to consult a veterinarian who is experienced in more than one type of therapy.

Although there is currently no clear explanation in Western scientific language as to how acupuncture works, there have been studies which help an understanding of it.

As recently as the 1970s it was discovered that the body can produce opium-like substances known as endorphins and enkephalins, whose properties resemble morphine in their ability to suppress pain. Numerous experiments have shown that the needling of acupuncture points stimulated the release of these substances into the bloodstream.

This is thought to be one of the reasons why putting a twitch on a horse works so effectively; the nose is a very tender area, and it seems strange that such an action, which should in principle cause tremendous pain, can result in a fractious animal standing calmly. However, if the twitch is putting pressure on an acupuncture

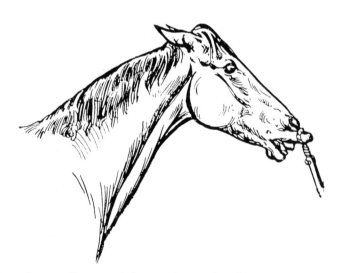

The calming influence of the twitch may be due to its pressure on acupuncture points, which stimulates the release of endorphins. The same technique is employed in the wild by pack animals to restrain their prey.

point, thus causing the release of endorphins, its success becomes more understandable. The principle is also demonstrated in the wild by pack animals, such as wild dogs, hunting their prey. One of their number will grasp the victim by the nose, which has the effect of quietening the animal, thus allowing the rest of the pack to carry on their grizzly business.

Such can be the power of these methods in relieving pain that major operations on humans have been carried out with no other anaesthesia than that provided by acupuncture.

Another theory is that the nervous system contains 'gates', which can open or close, to allow or prevent pain impulses passing to the brain. By stimulating pain inhibitory fibres through the use of acupuncture their effect is increased, causing a closing of the 'gate' for a period, thereby blocking the sensation of pain.

It is perhaps possible that acupuncture points may contain a greater proportion of the inhibiting nerve fibres; if these points are nerve-rich areas anyway, it would also explain how the immune system, which is partly under nervous control, can be affected, and how resistance to infection may be modified. However, these are very simplistic explanations.

Herbal medicine

There are many different systems of herbal medicine in use today. These are not conflicting in any way, but they do reflect the different cultures which have fostered the development of the philosophy. They all have one thing in common: the practitioner regards the patient as a whole, taking into consideration physical, environmental, and emotional circumstances. It was Hippocrates who said that herbal medicine is more of an art than a science, and as such its benefits may be appreciated more easily from a reflective than a definitive standpoint.

Pharmaceutical drugs differ from herbal medicines in several ways. Most importantly they are made of single chemical compounds, which are either isolated from plant extracts, or are synthetic copies or slightly altered models of plant extracts. They are purified so that the drug is available to the body in much higher doses.

Isolated extracts behave very differently from the way in which the whole plant behaves. For example, the foxglove contains cardioactive glycosides, which are widely used in treating heart conditions. Isolated single glycosides such as digitoxin are very useful, but their use is not without problems, because the effective medicinal dose is very close to the toxic dose. In the natural whole-plant extract, the glycosides are associated with other chemicals that control their availability. Because of this only one-tenth of the effective compound in the form of whole-plant extract is required in order to have the same effect on the heart as the glycosides in the purified drug. This means that the herbal medicine has the same effect with a lower risk.

Herbal medicines range across a wide spectrum. At one end dosage matters very little, and at the other, dosage is critical. Many herbs would not be regarded today as medicines: such things as garlic and liquorice are regularly eaten but not specifically for their medicinal qualities. In the middle ground are herbs such as the nervines – californian poppy and valerian, for instance – where the dose should be carefully chosen in relation to the individual symptoms. At the extreme end are the toxic herbs which must be used with great care. This is one of the reasons why horse-owners should only consult suitably qualified people.

It should be noted that membership of the British Herbal Medicines Association does not in itself enable the member to carry out treatment, as unqualified people can join. There are no recognised qualifications for veterinary herbalists, unlike human herbalists. It is illegal for non-veterinarians to prescribe or advise on herbal treatment, and failure to observe this can have legal consequences for the horse-owner too. As holistic medicine becomes more widely practised, there are an increasing number of veterinary surgeons prescribing herbal treatment.*

Before the rise of the modern pharmaceutical industry in the late 1950s and early 1960s, the study of drugs derived from plants, pharmacognosy, was part of the training for all medical students and those training as chemists. The main reason why these drugs fell out of favour has nothing to do with efficacy. Unlike herbs, modern drugs can be patented, and earn huge profits for the manufacturers every year. There is not much future from a

* More information is available from the BAHNM.

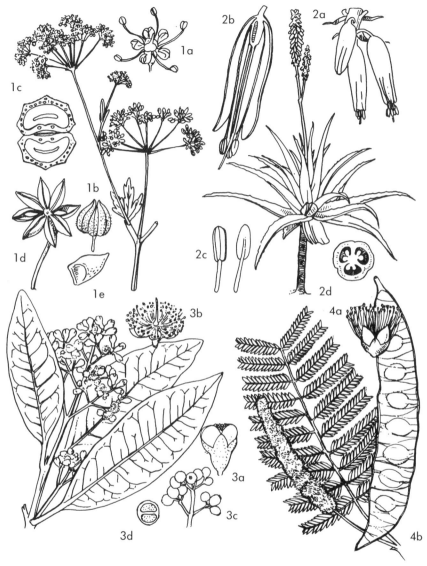

1. Aniseed (*Pimpinella anisum*): a. Flower enlarged. b. Fruit enlarged.
   c. Section across fruit. d. Star Aniseed (*Illicium verum*) partly open.
   e. Carpel.
2. Aloes, Barbados (*Aloe vulgaris*): a. Flower. b. Section of flower.
   c. Anthers. d. Section of ovary.
3. Red Pimento (*Pimenta officinalis*): a. Bud enlarged. b. Flower
   enlarged. c. Fruit. d. Cross section of fruit enlarged.
4. Catechu (*Acacia catechu*): a. Flower enlarged. b. Pod.

Some medicinal plants traditionally used in the treatment of horses.
Herbal medicine can be a safe and effective alternative to modern
drug therapy, provided that it is practised by qualified and suitably
experienced veterinarians. Some individual herbs may be used on a
regular basis for optimum nutrition, but the general use of unlicensed
poly-herbal feed additives is not recommended.

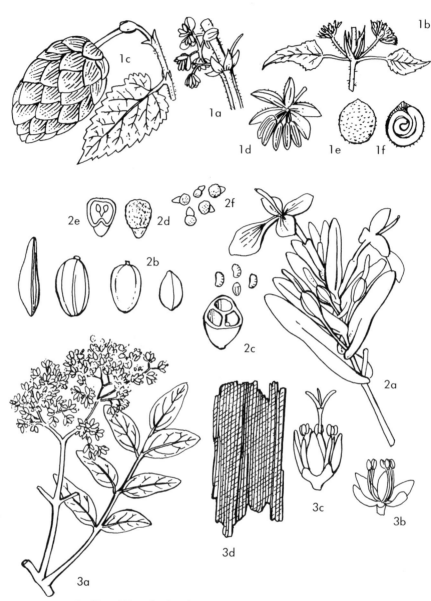

1. Hop (*Humulus lupulus*):
   a. Male flower. b. Female flower. c. Strobile. d. Male flower
   enlarged. e. Fruit enlarged. f. Section of fruit enlarged.
2. Cardamom (*Elettaria cardamomum*):
   a. Raceme. b. Cardamom. c. Section of fruit and seeds enlarged.
   d. Grain of Paradise (*Amomum melegarta*) enlarged. e. Section of
   Grain of Paradise. f. Section of seed, natural size.
3. Quassia (*Picraena excelsa*):
   a. Leaves and flowers reduced. b. Male flower enlarged.
   c. Hermaphrodite flower enlarged. d. Cross-grained slice of wood.

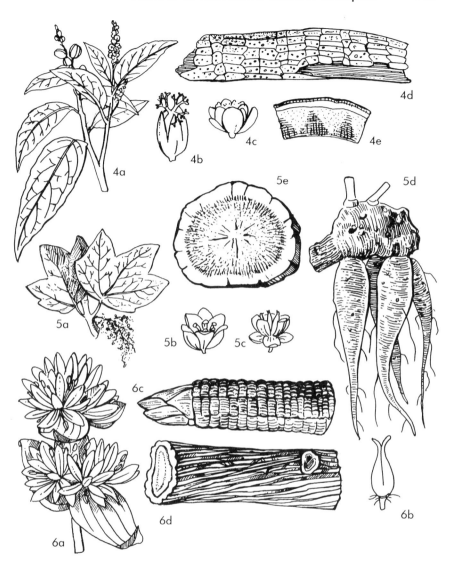

4. Cascarilla (*Croton eleuteria*):
   a. Branchlet. b. Female flower enlarged. c. Male flower enlarged.
   d. Bark. e. Cross section of bark enlarged.
5. Calumba (*Jateorhiza calumba*):
   a. Leaves and flowers reduced. b. Male flower enlarged.
   c. Female flower enlarged. d. Rhizome and roots reduced.
   e. Slice of root.
6. Gentian (*Gentiana lutea*):
   a. Upper part of flower spike. b. Fruit. c. Part of rhizome. d. Part
   of root.

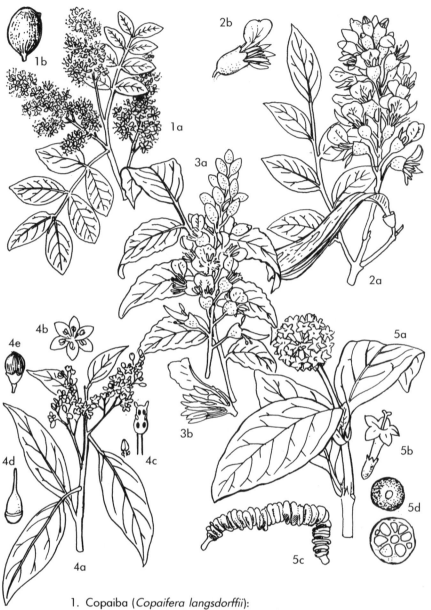

1. Copaiba (*Copaifera langsdorffii*):
   a. Plant reduced. b. Flower enlarged.
2. Balsam of Tolu (*Myroxylon toluifera*):
   a. Plant reduced. b. Flower, natural size.
3. Balsam of Peru (*Myroxylon pereiræ*):
   a. Plant reduced. b. Section of flower enlarged.
4. Camphor (*Laurus camphora*):
   a. Plant reduced. b. Flower enlarged. c. Stamina and staminodes
   enlarged. d. Pistil enlarged. e. Fruit.
5. Ipecacuanha (*Cephaëlis Ipecacuanha*):
   a. Plant. b. Flower enlarged. c. Root. d. Section of root
   enlarged.

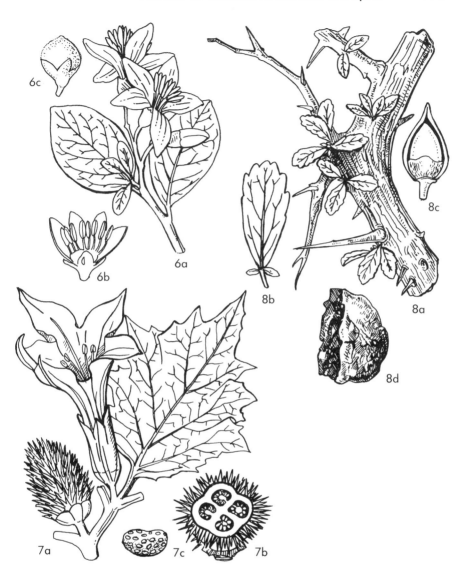

6. Storax (*Styrax officinale*):
   a. Plant.   b. Section of flower enlarged.   c. Fruit.
7. Stramonium (*Datura stramonium*):
   a. Plant reduced.   b. Section of fruit reduced.   c. Seed enlarged.
8. Myrrh (*Balsamodendron myrrha*):
   a. Plant.   b. Leaf enlarged.   c. Fruit with husk half-removed.
   d. Piece of myrrh.

marketing point of view to research and develop herbal medicines, which can then be copied by the competition, or grown by the consumer in the back garden. Far better to put money into researching a synthetic compound which would be patentable.

Largely because of this, the older, more established medical practices such as herbalism fell by the wayside, and pharmacognosy, the study of drugs derived from plants, was dropped by most educational institutions. Not only was herbal medicine in decline, but it was also ridiculed by the pharmaceutical industry, as well as by many members of the medical profession, who had become immersed in the new 'silver bullet' philosophy.

Although many modern drugs have saved countless lives, they cannot be said to be the miracle cures that everyone expected during the middle of the twentieth century. The modern scientific approach involves attempts to manipulate nature, which usually fail. For example, when we develop a product to destroy the causative organism of a particular disease, it will often mutate and continue its mission, rendering the product useless. This remarkable natural process happens quite spontaneously, making our progress in science seem like a novice against a Grand Master on the chess board. Furthermore, if we use drugs to counteract or suppress a bio-chemical process, the body will circumvent the blockade and the symptoms will return. The simple truth is that we must work with nature, rather than trying to cheat it. One of the strongest impulses in nature is the will of every organism to survive, but it will only be allowed to do so on the terms dictated by nature, not by mankind.

Another problem with synthetic products, apart from the fact that they usually only treat the symptoms, rather than the disease itself, is that they carry a risk of side effects. Although products are rigorously tested for 'safety, quality, and efficacy', there are still many risks involved, and countless horror stories to prove it.

Much of the testing is conducted in animal experiments, but this has inherent problems because of what is known as 'species difference'. The purifier of penicillin, Florey, said that it was a 'lucky chance' that he did not test it on guinea pigs; if he had the outcome would have been rather different, because it kills them very quickly. Despite the fact that the implications of this have been known for many years, mistakes are still being made; and a multitude of drugs passed as safe on animals have caused serious

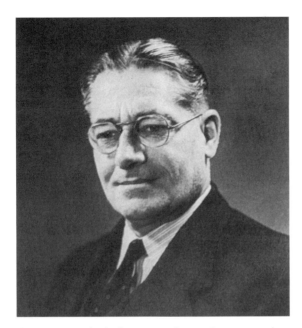

The way in which the same chemical compound can have different effects depending on the type of animal it is administered to is known as 'species difference'. Howard Florey, pictured above (c. 1940), quite by chance did not experiment on guinea pigs to develop and purify penicillin (he used other species). If he had, the outcome would have been rather different because it kills them very quickly. The principle of species difference also has many implications for the modern trend for poly-herbal products for horses, many of which are formulated by unsuitably qualified individuals using information gleaned from human herbals.

and even deadly side effects in humans.

There are now many more effective ways of testing synthetic products which do not involve vivisection. Methods such as cell tissue and organ culture are becoming more sophisticated. Not only are these new methods more relevant to the problem, and therefore safer, but they do not involve inhumanity to animals.

With synthetic products, we have made progress in conquering and controlling many diseases. Some of the antibiotics and chemical therapies for cancers have saved many lives, but we must keep them in the correct perspective. When used as a 'silver bullet', they can be remarkably effective in treating the symptoms of disease, and they are useful to keep in reserve. With an holistic approach, however, these products would be needed far less. Holistic veterinarians use a variety of methods which serve to avoid the need for such treatment, or at least to keep it to an absolute minimum. Some use holistic therapies so successfully that they rarely, if ever, use synthetic drugs of any kind.

Holistic medicine concentrates on the epidemiology of disease. It involves studying the cause of disease, its origins, and methods of spread. This knowledge enables preventive measures to be taken against many diseases. An example of this is how diet, stress, and exercise were shown to be connected with heart disease in humans. Epidemiology explained the way in which infectious diseases spread, by the discovery that isolated people could not pass them on. When disease is present, the holistic physician will endeavour to remove the barriers to healing, and the powerful natural healing process of the body can then begin, assisted if necessary by the various therapies which work in support of those processes.

As the routine use of many synthetic products falls out of vogue, along with the misplaced faith in the total ability of modern pharmaceutical products to heal everything, there is renewed interest in herbal medicine. Increasingly, pharmacognosy is being re-introduced to college courses for medical students.

All cultures have deep traditions of herbal medicines, and a study of those in different civilisations makes not only fascinating reading, but offers a wealth of medical lore. African tribes, North American Indians, Middle and Near Eastern cultures, the Indian subcontinent, the Far East, including of course China, Australian Aborigines, and many others show the wisdom of herbal medicine, and have a rich and diverse plant medicine culture deeply integrated into their societies. So widespread and varied are these botanical species that most people had easy access to plants with medical properties.

It is not surprising that our forefathers intermingled religion, folk-lore and superstition with their medicine. The power of the mind plays an important part in the healing process, and they knew it! Shamanism and its counterparts were linked to medical knowledge, and witch doctors, druids, tribal medicine men and later, in medieval Europe, the Christian Church became involved with medicine.

Astrology also became entangled with herbal medicine, a tradition epitomised by Nicholas Culpeper in the mid-seventeenth century.

Herbal medicine, however, holds its validity without the mystical and religious connotations handed down from ancient worlds. Sadly, however, many traditions of herbal medicine were unwritten and many formulae, enshrined in oral tradition, have been lost over the centuries as a result of the conquest of civilisations and the destruction of cultures. Many will not be rediscovered by our modern world. Even when records were made, wars and clashes of culture often combined to destroy them. For instance, 700,000 or more books amassed in the medical school in Alexandria, incorporating information from conquered territories such as India and the Middle East, were destroyed by Christian fanatics in 391 AD. In similar circumstances, the pictogram records of the Aztecs were destroyed by the Conquistadors.

Our Western herbal medicine culture dates back to Greek and Roman traditions, oversown with influences from medieval and other scholars through the ages, from all over Europe. Names such as Hippocrates, Pliny, Dioscorides, Galen, Paracelsus, Gerard, and Culpeper come up regularly in writings on the subject.

The rationale behind herbal medicine has changed as it has evolved. However, one recurring theme is the 'Doctrine of Signatures', which dates back to Paracelsus or even earlier. According to this principle, a plant could give a clue to its medical uses through its habitat, morphology and appearance. For example, *Chelidonium*, or Greater Celandine, is a remarkable remedy for jaundice. It led ancient prescribers to this idea through its having bright yellow sap, which turns skin a bright yellowy-orange on contact, exactly the colour of jaundiced skin. Turmeric was similarly adopted in the East. Nowadays, however, herbal medicines can be chosen because of their known medical properties through the action of their analysed ingredients. Active chemicals in plants, for example, alkaloids, glycosides, saponins, flavones etc., in unique combinations, have known medical effects explained by modern science. Herbs can be grouped according to their general action, for example, alteratives, aperients, astringents, bitters, demulcents, diuretics, expectorants, nervines, vulneraries etc. We will look at these in more detail below.

As we have seen, a great many modern conventional drug medicines are prepared from herbal materials, or at least have a herbal origin. Vincristine and vinblastine, which are two of the most effective modern treatments for cancers, started from the

Madagascar periwinkle. Aspirin, which is salicylic acid, may be obtained from willow or meadowsweet. Quinine, an effective treatment against malaria, is manufactured from the bark of a tree called cinchona. Digoxin, which is used in congestive heart failure, is from the foxglove. Morphine, a powerful pain-killer, comes from the opium poppy.

Many other drugs have originated from fungi: penicillin is from moulds; and ivermectin, which is a powerful anthelmintic and parasiticide, is from a soil fungus, to name but two. One major difference, however, between modern medicine and herbalism is the principle of holism. Holistic therapies treat the patient as a whole, rather than just the symptoms. They also use the medicines as a whole, by utilising the entire plant with its active medicinal ingredients and essential natural synergists.

One of the tragedies of modern times is that, just as we are beginning to take a serious scientific look at herbalism, one of the potential sources of material, the rain forests, is being destroyed. Many modern drugs developed against diseases such as glaucoma and cancers have been found amongst the cultures living in these areas, whose medicine men have been using them for generations. Over the last few decades we have seen the destruction of over half of the world's tropical rain forests, which are currently disappearing at an alarming rate. Research cannot keep up: they are disappearing faster than we can study them. One quarter of the drugs now regularly used in Western medicine originated in the rain forest. Despite this fact, only one per cent of rain forest plants have been studied adequately. There is a wealth of knowledge there, if we could tap into it; thousands of lives could be saved if we could redirect our resources in this direction, before they are lost forever.

Herbal medicine is admirably suited to the horse. As a herbivore his physiology is well adapted to benefit from plant material. Along with other herbivores, he has long been able to select instinctively his own natural medicine from the surrounding flora when given free access to a natural grazing environment. Horses may often be seen to dig for dandelion roots, for example, or other plants which we now know have a particular benefit.

Herbal medicine has been proved to be useful in treating the majority of diseases from which horses suffer. If herbal medicine is prescribed for your horse by a veterinarian practising holistic

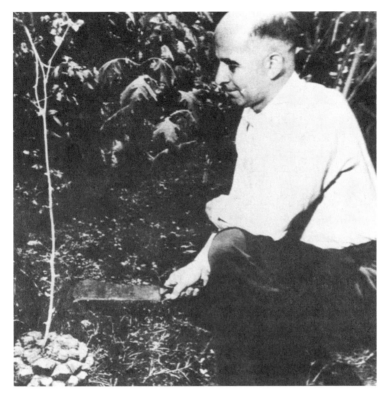

A great many modern drugs are either prepared from plants or have a plant origin. Russell Marker, pictured above in the early 1950s with a specimen of *Dioscorea*, developed progesterone from the natural product diosgenin found in the plant. One of the problems encountered with chemically altered natural compounds is the side effects they produce, which do not usually occur when the unadulterated herb is used.

medicine it will be as part of an integrated approach to healing. It may be used in conjunction with homoeopathy and acupuncture, and probably with dietary advice. Among the conditions that respond well are lung allergies, rheumatism and arthritis, hyper-excitability, digestive disorders and many others. Treatment with herbal medicine is without side-effects when used properly with regard to formulae and dosage. Instructions must be carefully followed. It can be given as dried herbage, capsules, powders, tinctures, infusions, oils and creams, and ointments.

It must be emphasised again that it is illegal for any person who is not a qualified veterinary surgeon to treat, or advise upon the treatment of, any disease or condition of animals. Thus the detailed information on herbs and their uses given below must not encourage the horse-owner to diagnose and treat disease. Many of the herbs listed here are toxic, and should only be used by those qualified to do so. However, some of them may be used as regular feed additives. Owners are recommended to take proper and legally qualified advice regarding their suitability and dosage.

In addition if the horse is being given herbal remedies and requires further veterinary attention, it is wise to consult an holistic veterinary surgeon, or at least one who understands the interactions of herbs and drugs.

Categories of herbs

Herbs are divided into categories, depending on their action on the body. Specific combinations of herbs will produce different effects depending on the circumstances, and on the food being consumed, which makes herbalism a fascinating study.

Individual herbs are chosen both for their action and the degree of action. Oak bark, for instance, is a strong astringent, but varying degrees of astringency are available from tormentiel and ribwort.

As with other types of holistic therapy, herbal medicine sees the symptoms as part of a larger problem. Thus constipation may be treated with herbs to stimulate liver action and bile production. Eczema would not be seen simply as a rash to be treated, but herbs to encourage the natural cleansing system of the body would be used. This approach is sometimes difficult to understand without a working knowledge of the principles involved.

Alteratives

Alteratives act on the metabolism, helping it to progress normally. They are used in conjunction with the depuratives, otherwise known as blood cleansers. Many plants can have this effect on the system, but they achieve it in different ways. The types chosen reflect the overall symptoms and causes of the problem. Alteratives work by supporting the role of the blood in collecting and dumping the waste material from the liver and kidneys. The alterative herbs work on the lymphatic system which, as part of this elimination process, bathe the cells of the body, removing waste material for subsequent elimination. The alteratives are particularly useful when the immune system may be compromised in some way. Associated conditions which may indicate the use of alteratives are: eczema, inflammation of the joints, swollen lymph glands, and tumours.

Antimicrobial, antiseptic, anti-infective

All these are aimed at keeping infective organisms at bay. There are many herbs available with suitable properties. As well as using medicines to attack the organisms themselves, the holistic practitioner will use medicines to strengthen the body's own defence mechanisms.

The immune system is central to the ability of the body to fight off disease. Associated with this process is the production of white blood cells, which are the defensive army of the body. If the immune system is working properly, the white blood cells and antibodies will attack and destroy any invading organism. This is possible through a complex system which enables the white cells to recognise and act against alien cells, whilst ignoring those which are not alien. A number of factors can compromise the immune system, such as the many synthetic products given to horses in feeds and supplements. Constant use of these products over-load the system, throwing it out of balance, thereby reducing the effectiveness of the mechanism. The anti-infective herbs work by strengthening the immune system.

Antispasmodics

Antispasmodics are used to relax the muscles, when this is thought to be beneficial by the practitioner. Muscle spasm happens in response to many situations, and is the body's natural protective mechanism at work. After injury, for instance, the muscles controlling the affected part will go into painful spasm, preventing further use. If these spasms continue for any reasons that are not beneficial to the situation, anti-spasmodics may be used to relax the system and release the tension in the affected muscles. This promotes a return to a normal blood flow through the affected part, which is an integral part of the body's own healing process. Many horses suffer from nervous tension at some time, which can affect performance and health. Because antispasmodics are in effect relaxants, they are particularly useful in treating management problems associated with stress. They are also beneficial in the treatment of stress-related physiological problems such as poor digestion.

Anti-inflammatory

Inflammation occurs in the body for good reason, as part of the normal healthy response to irritation, injury, or infection. The inflammation is a sign that the body is responding appropriately, allowing circumstances around the site of the problem to change in order to facilitate healing. Swelling is a result of dilation of blood vessels, which allows more blood to flow around the area, providing the required agents for the healing process and effusion of fluids into the tissues. This causes certain other changes: pain and redness, caused by increased local blood flow, and heat caused by increased metabolic activity. The inflammation is seen as a good sign that the body's mechanisms are working well, and progress is compared to the cause. The body may need some support in dealing with the underlying problem, and this may be treated simultaneously. Most of the herbs used as anti-inflammatories actually work by speeding up or modulating the inflammatory process rather than suppressing it. This may be done using bitters, volatile oils or herbs containing sesquiterpine lactones.

Anti-tussives and expectorants

A cough is a reflex action of the throat to expel unwanted material from the respiratory tract. The cough is a natural action of the body, responding appropriately to a stimulus. Coughing is of great concern to horse-owners. Often it is connected with stabling conditions, such as bedding or feed, with environmental conditions, such as pollen allergy, or has a deeper significance. Coughing is a useful mechanism if it is cleansing: however, unproductive dry coughs may not be seen by the practitioner as beneficial. In these circumstances an anti-tussive may be used to soothe the cough reflex.

An expectorant works on the respiratory tract by softening and helping to dislodge phlegm and mucus. This may then be expelled from the system through the cough mechanism. It follows that anti-tussives and expectorants are rarely used together.

The expectorants may be divided into two categories which describe their method of action: relaxants and stimulants. The stimulating expectorants encourage the small hairs, or cilia, in the respiratory tract to move phlegm and mucus to the top of the respiratory tract, so that it can then be either swallowed or expelled. The relaxing expectorants soothe the muscle spasms and soften the phlegm deep within the lungs. When using expectorants the problem often appears to get worse before it gets better. This is because the phlegm and mucus must be removed before the healing process can begin.

Bitters

Bitters are important in many areas of medicine. Their main target areas in the body are the liver and the digestive system. The liver is often referred to as the most important chemical processing plant of the body. It has many important parts to play. It is involved in the production of usable proteins, the building blocks of the body; it controls the circulation of important substances, such as sugars; it acts as a storage area for glycogen and for fat-soluble vitamins; and it breaks down waste for subsequent elimination through the system. The digestive system involves several processes involving the chemical changes required to assimilate food into the body as useful nutrients. Many factors can effect this process and the chemical balance of the system must be maintained for it to function properly.

Bitters may be used in conditions where the function of the liver or gall bladder has been reduced. Bitters are used to stimulate the liver to produce bile, which is then stored in the gall bladder to be released into the system as required. The secretion of bile into the system can be stimulated by the use of mountain grape (*Berberis aquifolium*) and celandine (*Chelidonium majus*), for example.

Carminatives

Carminatives act on the digestive tract. They calm and relieve flatulence and other symptoms which may lead to colic. The ones most used are generally rich in volatile oils, such as spices.

Demulcents and emollients

Herbs in this category are used to provide mucilage, which soothes and softens the surfaces with which it comes into contact. They are commonly used to protect irritated or inflamed mucus membranes in the throat, and other areas of the digestive and urinary systems. They are also used in the treatment of skin conditions to relieve irritation.

Uterine and menstrual

Many of these herbs, together with the hormonal herbs, are used for mares where there is a connection between unbalanced temperament and the oestrus cycle. They are particularly effective and must be used with great care, especially during pregnancy. They are directed specifically towards the uterus and associated organs. Some of the herbs used are stimulants, and others relaxants. The choice of which to use depends on the diagnosis and the required effect in the light of other factors.

Hormonal herbs
Many hormonal herbs are used in conjunction with uterine and menstrual herbs. Their action is to affect the endocrine glands, which are associated with hormonal problems. These include the pituary, thyroid, adrenal, ovaries, testes, and pancreas. There are a multitude of herbs in this category available to the practitioner which may affect one or all of these glands depending upon the desired result.

Vulneraries or wound healers
There are many herbs which may be used for this purpose, depending upon the type and location of the wound. Weeping wounds can be effectively treated with astringents, infection can be reduced with other herbs. Some can be used to draw the two sides of a wound together, and others to provide a protective coating. Comfrey is widely used for its healing powers. It contains the chemical allantoin, which speeds the repair process of damaged tissue.

Homoeopathy

Homoeopathy was the brainchild of Samuel Hahnemann, a German physician who in the late eighteenth century developed a system of medicine which exploits the natural reaction of the body to an external stimulus in order to bring about a healing effect. It is developed from two basic theories that 'like cures like' and 'less is more'.

The word homoeopathy comes from the Greek '*homoios*' and '*pathos*', meaning 'similar sickness'. Hahnemann had qualified as a physician by the time he was twenty-four, having paid for his training out of the proceeds of translating medical books into German from several languages. He began looking for more enlightened forms of medicine than those of the day, which included many crude practices such as blood letting, and which used medicines of a suppressive or even downright dangerous nature. He began to study further and returned to his translating work and to chemistry for a living. It was during this work that he came across quinine, an accepted anti-malarial drug, and a remarkable sequence of events began.

His first experiments to find how the drug worked were performed with the parent material of quinine. He found that it produced in himself symptoms which were quite indistinguishable from malaria. He felt that he had discovered the principle of cure by 'similars', which had been alluded to by Hippocrates in his fourth century BC writings.

A research team in the United States led by Mathew Kluger has put forward a theory which coincides with Hahnemann's theory of 'similars'. Kluger's theory was that the body's natural way of dealing with infection, for instance, was to raise the temperature, increasing the mobility of the white blood cells, which are part of the body's defence system. It also increases the body's ability to produce the chemical interferon, which is effective against viruses. The modern medical approach would be to lower the fever, and while this should be done in certain circumstances the value of the fever itself should be considered. It may be that we should aid and modulate the fever, not suppress it. Many modern medicines work in opposites; if we have a headache we take a pain killer, when what we should be doing is looking at the reasons for the headache and seeking a method of balancing the body to help it remove disease.

By meticulous and surprisingly scientific experiments on himself and other healthy volunteers, Hahnemann discovered that a substance can cure a disease with a particular set of symptoms, if it is able to produce a similar set of symptoms in a healthy body. He continued his work in many areas of disease and developed a huge range of homoeopathic medicines which followed the principle of like curing like. We now have several thousand remedies.

In 1810, Hahnemann published his philosophy and findings in a book called *The Organon of the Healing Art*, which is the foundation stone for the principle today. Homoeopathy became fashionable in America around the mid 1800s. Many famous people supported the practice, including Mark Twain and Louisa May Alcott.

Hahnemann developed a second principle, which has led to

incredulity from the modern scientific medical community. He found that serial dilution and succussion (violent shaking) of the substances produced not only safer medicines but more powerfully effective ones. This is only explicable in energy terms, since Hahnemann's dilutions were often so extreme as to be sub-molecular in concentration.

The acceptance of homoeopathy in different parts of the world varied. In the United States the conventional, or allopathic, medical community started by outlawing the practice, as often occurs when something new appears. It happens for a variety of reasons, but it is a reaction not justifiable on technical grounds alone. Homoeopathy is now accepted by the American Medical Association, which, incidentally, was formed some years later than the American Institute of Homoeopathy. The practice is widespread in Europe, but is still regarded with suspicion, and no doubt fear, by the medical establishment in some countries.

In England, homoeopathy flourishes, helped along initially by royal patronage. The royal family set a trend which is now firmly established, rather surprisingly, given the phlegmatic attitude of the nation toward anything new. By 1977 there were six National Health hospitals providing homoeopathy, and they served 86,000 people as out-patients. Homoeopathic medicines are freely available through chemists and other outlets.

Despite its efficacy and widespread acceptance there are still attempts to debunk homoeopathy on the grounds that it cannot be properly explained in terms which suit the allopathic medical establishment. Recently, dramatic evidence of the efficacy of homoeopathy was substantiated by 'double blind trials'. These are standard tests used in modern medicine where the effects of a drug are tested by giving the real drug to some patients and an inert substance to others. It is called a double blind trial because neither the patients nor the doctors know which substance is being used. In these trials there was remarkable evidence to show that the homoeopathic medicines were effective, but the official mainstream medical bodies still chose either to ignore them or to dismiss them out of hand. Accusations were made against the medical publications at the time, claiming reports were slanted firmly against homoeopathy. So much for open-mindedness.

That Hahnemann was able to cure hitherto untreatable diseases was a revelation in itself. That he was able to do so without harmful side effects was an amazing development. However, his dilutions discovery served to alienate homoeopathy from the established conventional medicine of the day. Hahnemann discovered that the more he diluted the medicines, the safer and more powerful they became.

Homoeopathy is classed as an 'energy medicine'. It operates directly on the dynamic and energetic processes of the body, modulating and harmonising its daily workings and restoring normal function. It can create no residue, which makes homoeopathy very popular with the competition horse's owner.

The fact that the medicines work by harmonising the body's processes means that an artificially stimulated performance cannot be achieved, only optimum performance; so homoeopathic medicine is totally acceptable, morally and ethically. Pregnant mares may also be safely treated with no risk of harming the unborn foal.

Conditions that respond to homoeopathic treatment are spread across the entire spectrum of equine ailments: acute problems such as injury, sprains, fractures, equine influenza and viruses, and wound infections, and chronic conditions such as sinusitis, laminitis, sweet itch, COPD, spavin, arthritis, navicular, and other degenerative bone diseases.

The method of selection of a homoeopathic medicine follows holistic principles; the whole body, its life-style, environment and management is taken into account. The whole body includes the mind, so mental symptoms, demeanour, and behaviour are very important in formulating the best therapy.

Medicines are chosen according to the pattern of disease and its characteristics within a particular patient, as opposed to selection according to the name of the disease. For this reason a given homoeopathic medicine can be effective in a great many different conditions whose symptoms match the medicine. Equally a disease may be treated by any one of a great number of different homoeopathic medicines, selected according to the particular symptoms displayed by the patient.

This tailoring of the treatment to the individual explains the great success of homoeopathy when correctly applied, but it can also be the cause of great confusion and difficulty for the inexperienced prescriber. One of the reasons for this is that modern science teaches the philosophy of treating one problem with one drug, which is alien to the theory of holism.

Osteopathy, chiropractic

medicine, and like many other complementary therapies are now available for the horse. It is, of course, of special importance to keep the musculo-skeletal system of the horse in good order, and these therapies are designed to do this. Therapist in this area, like other non-veterinary practitioners, must work within the confines of the Veterinary Surgeons Act 1966, which makes it illegal for non-veterinary surgeons to treat a disease or condition. They may, however, work under the auspices of a veterinary surgeon within strict guidelines.

Manipulative therapy has been in use for at least 2000 years. There are Greek records which explain how legs could be manoeuvred to ease problems of the lower back. Hippocrates wrote of the importance of the spine in relation to diseases of limbs and muscles. Ancient cultures employed children to walk along the backs of adults to relieve pain and help flexibility. One amusing story involved Captain Cook, the famous explorer, while he was in Tahiti in the late 1700s. He complained to the local chieftain of the back pains which were troubling him, and several rather large women were sent to his ship on a number of occasions to administer a treatment. This consisted of pulling and pushing his body in all directions, which, according to his ship's log, often produced loud cracking noises. Apparently, after several visits, he began to feel much better.

Chiropractic

The central function is the alignment of the spinal column, which can be connected with many other conditions of the skeletal and nervous system. This often includes manipulation of other parts of the body, depending upon the approach of the practitioner. Like other holistic therapies it works to keep the body in harmony and balance by regularising the skeletal and muscular systems. More particularly, it has an effect on the segmental nervous system by removing tensions on the nerves as they emerge from the spine.

Osteopathy

Osteopathy was created by a man called Andrew Still in the United States, during the Civil War. Typical of many developers of alternative therapies he despaired of the practices of medicine carried out in his day. He could see little benefit from the common practices of bleeding with leeches and purging. What led him to this new way of thinking about how the skeletal and muscular framework could be implicated in disease was remembering how he could often cure his own headaches by cracking bones in his neck. The method of manipulation that he used was one of leverage and torsion, working on a low velocity, high amplitude manipulation.

Chiropractic came a little later than osteopathy, around 1895. A man called Daniel David Palmer, having investigated the new techniques of osteopathy, decided to advance his own, slightly different theory, while still agreeing with the basic principle. Chiropractic is now a prevalent form of manipulation in horses, utilising a high velocity, low amplitude manipulation. The manipulative force is usually applied directly to the offending area, and consists of very small, sudden and powerful adjusting movements, usually with the hands.

In either case, the therapist works to identify areas where the musculo-skeletal system is out of alignment. This is obviously very important in the general health and well-being of the horse, and many behavioural and physical problems can arise from misalignments. Stresses and strains are placed on the frame of the horse, particularly his back, when he is carrying a rider. Obviously this is compounded in athletic activities such as jumping. Whilst the skill and balance of the rider are of paramount importance here, the soundness of the horse's basic physiology and anatomy is a prerequisite to good health.

Any activity which makes the horse uncomfortable will be obvious to the observant rider. There may be a number of causes, and problems involving the musculo-skeletal and nervous system will be considered by the veterinarian, along with other possible causes. If a back or pelvic problem is found, it could have developed for a number of reasons, for example from a previous fall, a badly fitting saddle, a slip or badly co-ordinated movement, or a combination of all these. Often horses are labelled 'ungenerous' when they are unwilling to give of their best in certain circumstances; it is more likely, however, that they are in some discomfort or pain elicited by that particular activity.

If manipulative therapy is prescribed by the veterinarian, what the therapist is seeking to do is to return the musculo-skeletal and nervous system back to normal. This is done by looking for any areas of the body that are out of alignment; then by one or the other system, encouraging the misalignment back into place.

Areas in the spine and pelvis that are out of alignment are referred to as subluxations. These may have an effect on the normal functioning of the nerves associated with them. When they are back into alignment, the body's natural system of integration is resumed. As with all holistic therapies, the best results are obtained when the therapy is used in conjunction with preventative management. This will include saddling and riding considerations.

Radionics

Like many complementary therapies which have been successfully used on humans beings, radionics is now being used more frequently on animals. It is interesting that the success rate in using radionics therapy is slightly higher in animals than in human beings.

An American neurologist, Albert Abrams, was involved in early experiments which led later researchers to develop the theory of radionics. He discovered that the human abdomen could be used as a diagnostic sounding board. This technique, still practised today, involves the use of the fingers of one hand being placed flat against the abdomen, and then tapped with the tips of the fingers of the other hand. The resulting noise, either dull or hollow, could be related to diseased tissue. He concluded that the sound waves or energy being produced was a direct reflection of the condition of the organ. He took this further, and reproduced similar changes in energy patterns in various experiments involving the use of diseased cadavers being connected to healthy patients through wires. He noted that different diseases caused different patterns of energy, and interestingly the experiments were affected by the position of the patients in relation to the earth's magnetic field.

By painstaking research he was able to measure the electrical effect that the different experiments were producing in terms of ohms (an accepted scientific measurement of electrical resistance). Having related this measurable energy, or vibration, to the diagnosis of various diseases, Abrams believed that there was a potential for using these forces as a cure. Up until then he had only been using human beings in his experiments, largely for developing a diagnostic technique.

He hit on the idea of trying to build a machine that would simulate the body's energy, which could then be used to treat disease. A talented scientist and technician, Samuel Hoffmann, worked with Abrams and together they developed a machine called the oscilloclast. This was an electrically powered device which could direct varying vibrational patterns to the inner organs of the body, through an electrode placed on the patient's skin.

The treatment with the oscilloclast involved several sessions of up to an hour. However, considerable success was being achieved. Although treatment with such a machine seems crude by comparison to the radionics techniques used today, the principle of treating disease using this energy force was established.

Radionics is based on the theory that all forms of life are surrounded by a life-force or energy pattern, which radiates from within; this may be likened to a kind of magnetic field. It is now widely accepted that some kind of force-field exists, however we might like to explain it.

These energy fields are individual to each organism, rather like finger prints or DNA. They are reflective of the owner's state of health, and diseases are represented as changes within the fields. It may be thought of as a kind of radar scanning of the organism, though this is a very simplistic analogy. Various methods of analysis and therapy are employed by first taking a blueprint of the energy field of the organism. The blueprint is taken by using a small sample of blood, or piece of hair from the patient. This is called the 'witness', which is then placed in an apparatus which will register the pattern and strength of the energy waves being emitted. This apparatus is sometimes known as the 'black box'.

Radionic therapy is based on the principle that these force fields alter when the body is out of balance. This may happen for a variety of reasons, and the imbalance may be slight or dramatic. Imbalances may be the indicators of physical problems and consequently are related to disease. In common with many holistic therapies, radionics is less concerned with the actual disease symptoms than with seeing them as an indicator of an overall imbalance.

The equipment used in radionic therapy is designed to help the practitioner to identify the particular area of disease, and then change the pattern of it by redressing the energy waves. This can be done from considerable distances. The way the energy is transmitted over long distances may be compared to the principle of radio waves, which is done through a transmitter and a receiver.

This equipment is some way removed from the oscilloclast developed by Abrams, but the principle of harnessing energy and using it as part of a healing therapy remains. By comparison with many other therapies radionics is a comparatively new science and there is much to be learned, although remarkable advances have been made in the field over the last few years. New ideas and techniques are being developed which make the application of the basic theory more sophisticated and effective.

Radionics practitioners are able to work at great distances from their patients, which raises levels of scepticism in doubters. This remoteness, however, makes it an easy system to abuse by a disreputable practitioner. Be sure to check up on the credentials and reputation of those that you ask to do this work for you. Furthermore, be wary of accepting medicines sent out by practitioners, since this practice is illegal under the Veterinary Surgeons Act. Radionics is a diagnostic tool which can also 'treat' remotely, and does not involve the sending of medicines.

Magnet therapy

Magnet therapy is becoming increasingly popular as a method of treatment for horses. It is an old-established therapy which attracted interest in the 1950s in Japan. Several magnetic instruments have gained approval from the United States licensing authority, the Food and Drug Administration. Treatment consists of applying magnetic pads to the body, and the theory of the treatment is that the magnetic energy of the pads beneficially affects the cells and tissues.

Bio-magnetics has been used successfully for over forty years in the treatment of certain types of fractures, where other procedures have failed. Experiments have revealed that there are a number of physiological processes which may be affected by magnetic fields. For example, separate independent clinical trials have clearly shown the ability of bio-magnetics to increase the flow of blood.

There are several theories on how the magnetic fields of the body are related to those of the earth, and there has been plenty of scientific research in this area. A significant amount was carried out during the course of space research by the US space agency NASA. There are thought to be very significant differences in the effects on the body of the magnetic fields of the South and North Poles of the earth. It is believed that the South Pole stimulates the body's physiology, and the North Pole sedates it. Conclusions drawn from this research with regard to the relation between polarities and disease are that the normal healthy body is in a negatively polarised state.

It has been found that cells lose their polarity as a result of injury, which impairs their function. Bio-magnetic therapy returns the cells to normal polarity and metabolism. There are obviously many applications for the use of the therapy in the treatment of horses. As a holistic therapy, bio-magnetics is often used in conjunction with other disciplines, such as nutrition.

The therapy has been successfully used in the relief of pain and inflammation, to stimulate tissues, and to increase circulation of blood and oxygen. These actions are of particular benefit where the removal of stored toxins is required as part of the treatment.

Physiotherapy

A significant degree of help is provided for horses by physiotherapy, which is an aid to restoration of normal muscular function by controlled movement. Massage, manipulation of limbs, stimulation of muscles by Faradic machines, ultrasound therapy etc. all serve to increase circulation, remove toxins and aid healing. However, this is not a system of medicine in its own right and should only be used as an adjunct to the correction of medical and physical problems by acupuncture, herbal medicines, homoeopathy or chiropractic work. Used in this way by properly qualified and sensitive practitioners it can have tremendous benefits for the horse who is in the rehabilitation phase of disease or injury.

Posture training

The Greeks defined the principles of classical riding techniques some two thousand years ago. They understood how the rider could interfere with the horse's natural balance and co-ordination.

Posture is the most important element of self-carriage, and good posture is central to balanced riding. The way that the horse is ridden is directly related to the potential for problems involving the musculo-skeletal system. Owing largely to our modern sedentary life-style there is a decrease in back suppleness and self support, and this is reflected in riding posture.

Modern schools of thought have tended to concentrate on either the balance of the horse, or the balance of the rider. The classical ideal is to attain a perfect balance of the two. This involves a fluidity of movement which some riders seem to possess instinctively and others have to learn. It involves an understanding of the principles of movement and balance of both horse and rider.

The principles of good posture require effort, particularly at first and if the body is used to poor posture. Correct posture, both when standing and when sitting on a horse, will be naturally assumed providing the basic principles are followed.

One method, the Alexander Technique, is currently receiving much attention. The technique concentrates on achieving a better balance between horse and rider by improving the poise and posture of the rider. Strictly speaking it is a therapy for the rider rather than the horse, but the rider transfers the effects of the technique to the horse, with a beneficial outcome.

The Alexander Technique is based on the comparatively recent insights of Frederick Alexander who discovered that the position of the head and neck in relation to the rest of the body is crucial to overall co-ordination and efficient locomotion. His insights into these issues paralleled the theories of the Greeks centuries earlier.

Alexander came to London from his native Australia in 1904, and began to teach others the techniques of the therapy that he had taught himself. He taught many people, including Aldous Huxley and Bernard Shaw, until his death in 1955. Some twenty years before his death he started training courses to instruct others how to teach his work.

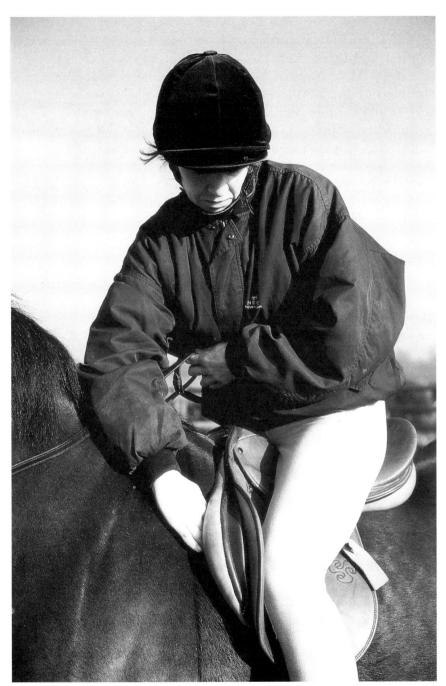

Correct saddle fitting is central to the horse's comfort and welfare. The potential for physical problems developing will be greatly reduced by regular attention to this vital but often neglected requirement.

The Alexander method of working is almost always taught individually, and the lesson depends very much on the needs of the pupil at the time. Essentially, the teacher has to change the way that the pupil uses his or her body. This is done by developing an attitude of not trying too hard to achieve results, but to take the time to think about how the results are to be achieved.

The teacher works with his hands on the pupil, not in a manipulative way, or anything like massage, but rather a gentle guiding of the musculature into a new poised, light, balanced state.

While this may take a little practice at first, it becomes a habit; bringing many benefits, such as improved breathing, less physical strain, and improved co-ordination and balance.

Saddlery and tack

The horse's way of going is also directly and crucially related to saddlery and tack, although this is not strictly a therapy. Having corrected one's own poise and control it is necessary to transmit clear unequivocal signals to the horse. These only need to be gentle commands if horse and rider are in harmony. For them to be transmitted correctly, however, bridle and bit must be correctly selected and adjusted for the horse. Saddlery must be comfortable and safe, both for horse and rider. It is comparatively easy for a rider to assess his or her own comfort in the saddle, but less easy to understand or to obtain help for arranging correct saddling for horses. Sadly, all too often it is not achieved and the suffering and disease which follow are a severely underestimated tragedy. Many harnessing aids are employed to try forcibly to correct wrong posture in horses which is actually the result of bad saddling. Far from helping, these methods can exacerbate the problems for the horse because they disallow the pain-avoidance responses.

Correct saddling theory is beyond the scope of this book but do not misjudge its central importance to the health and welfare of the horse.*

* Guidance on correct saddling can be obtained through the BAHNM.

7

Fitness

'Sound in wind and limb.'

The condition of the respiratory organs, together with the general condition of the body, and in particular the limbs, are central to the fitness of the horse. Consideration of the basic function of these systems and how they are interrelated gives an insight into their importance in general management.

The musculo-skeletal system

The musculo-skeletal system of the horse takes a great deal of strain when the horse is ridden, particularly during strenuous exercise and in competitive events. An appreciation of the anatomy of the skeleton and the principles of mechanics is a prerequisite for sympathetic riding.

The skeleton itself is the basic framework of the body. It is articulated by various types of joints, which are held together and motivated by a system of tendons, ligaments and muscles. It is an extremely strong structure which is not easily damaged during normal activities. However, when the horse is ridden special consideration must be given to the way the system works, so that it is not damaged.

Locomotion is made possible through the action of the muscles on the bones, which is a series of lever actions. The muscles involved in this process are mostly attached to the respective bones, either directly or through tendons. A lever is a rigid bar used to move objects by means of a fulcrum. The position of the

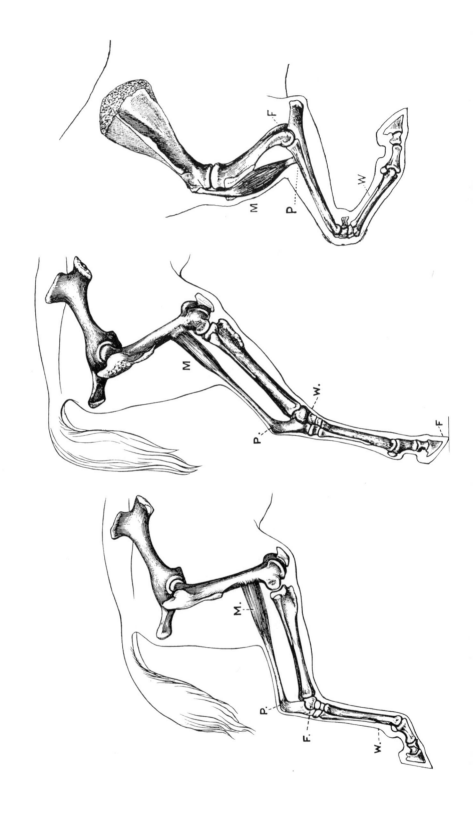

fulcrum along the bar has a significant effect on the ability of the lever to move various weights.

When a bone is operating as a lever, part of it is 'fixed' within a joint, and the other end moves in the required direction. A lever has three elements: the fulcrum, the power, and the weight. The efficiency of the lever in terms of development of force and speed depends on the relation of the power to the weight.

There are three kinds of levers, and it can be seen from the diagrams how these operate. The first kind of lever is one where the fulcrum is placed between the power and the load, as illustrated in the action of a pair of scales. This kind of lever is usually concerned with speed, as on p. 136 (*left*). Here the extension of the cannon on the hock can be seen, when the foot is off the ground. The muscle above the hock, which is the power, acts upon the point of the hock which is the fulcrum, moving the part below, which is the weight.

The second kind of lever is where the fulcrum is situated at one end, and the power is at the other, with the load in between, as illustrated by a person pushing a wheelbarrow. There are fewer levers of this kind in the skeleton, and they are essentially involved with force as on p. 136 (*centre*). Here the point of the hock is where the power acts, the weight is at the hock joint, and the ground is the fulcrum. Bones which act as levers of the first kind when the foot is off the ground become levers of the second kind when the foot is on the ground, the fulcrum and the load having changed places.

The third kind of lever is where the load is at one end, the fulcrum is at the other end, and the power is in the middle. An example of this is the action of lifting a load with a shovel. Levers of this kind are also involved with speed, but usually employed to flex limbs, as on p. 136 (*right*). Here the fulcrum is at the elbow joint, the power is the bicep muscle, and the weight is the limb below.

(Opposite) The principles of leverage operating in the bones of the legs of the horse. F Fulcrum P Point at which the power acts W Weight M Muscle which is the source of power. The design and action of the horse's legs reflects his evolved reliance upon speed to evade predators (and also the ability to deliver a powerful kick when appropriate). Strain on the legs is obviously increased under the weight of the rider, and is greatly amplified during competitive sports such as eventing, where fitness and good horsemanship are of paramount importance in preventing injury.

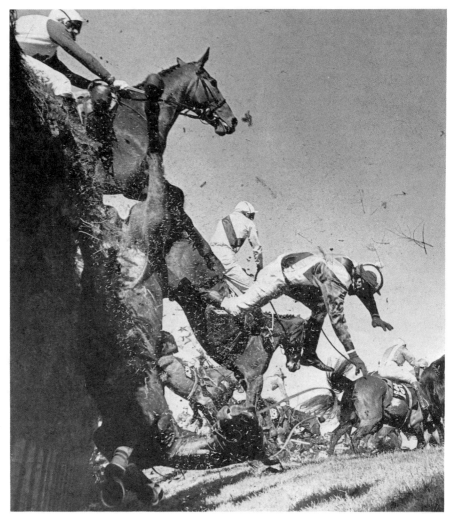

Brown Trix (nearest) broke his shoulder on landing, and both he and Seeandem, who is out of the picture, had to be destroyed. Despite the thrill of racing many find the risks involved in this kind of event too high for both horses and riders.

Detailed study of the principles and working of the levers in relation to the joints will provide an insight into the mechanical strains involved when working a horse in particular disciplines. Imagine, for instance, the strain imposed on the bones and ligaments of the horse's front feet when landing from a big jump with a rider aboard, or the opposing forces placed on the hock joints when negotiating complicated multiple jumps at advanced eventing level.

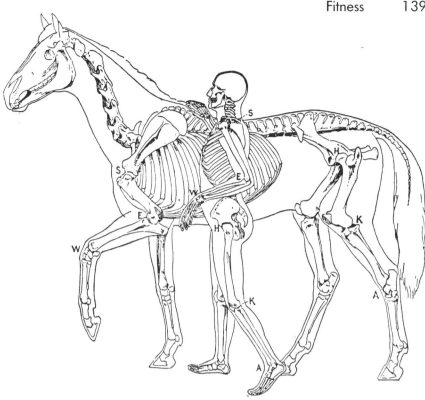

Comparative view of skeletons of man and horse. S Shoulder joint E
Elbow joint W Wrist joint (so-called knee in the horse) H Hip joint K
Knee (stifle joint in horse) A Ankle (hock joint in horse). Evolution has
modified the skeletal structure of each species. Although there are
differences between both the size and the shape of bones, joint articu-
lations have much in common. Some joints in man, such as the wrist
and ankle, have the additional capability of rotational movement as
well as flexion and tension.

Horses are athletic animals by nature, but they are not essentially
designed to jump off the ground, let alone when carrying a rider.
Comparison of the horse's anatomy with that of a creature which
is designed to jump gives an indication of the principles involved.
Creatures which are designed to jump, such as the frog, possess
elongated limbs and well-developed muscles in order to produce
the required leverage. Consideration of the mechanical principles
shown above and overleaf (*top*) gives an idea of the comparative
effort required by the horse when jumping.

Of course, horses can and do jump most effectively, and jumping
can undoubtedly be enjoyed by both horse and rider. However,

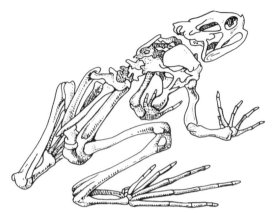

Skeleton of the frog. The legs of animals which have been adapted for jumping are proportionally larger than the legs of animals which are principally designed for running. The frog is capable of propelling itself into the air to a level which is many times its own height. It can be appreciated what energy is required of the horse to lift itself and the rider over even relatively small jumps.

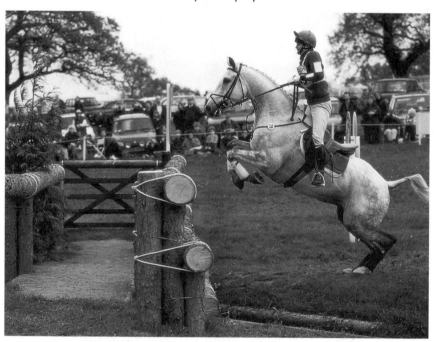

Although the horse is no longer the main means of transport and power, his athletic potential and conformation is being preserved through breeding and training for modern competition sports such as eventing. If these sports are to be performed without unacceptable risks of injury, fitness and rider skill are essential.

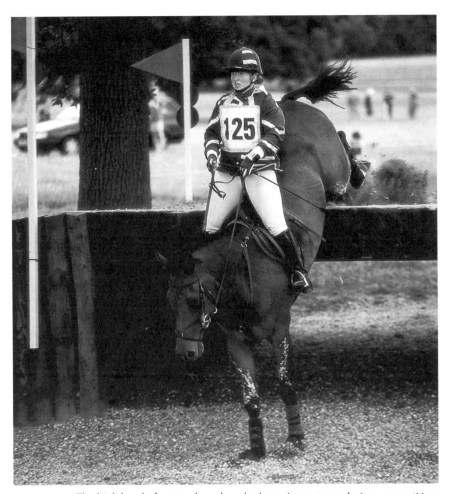

The high level of stress placed on the horse's anatomy during competition work means that long training is required to achieve and maintain appropriate strength and fitness. The importance of this can be appreciated here where the combined weight of horse and rider is being taken on the front legs of the horse. While this is only for a fraction of a second, there is tremendous strain on the tendons and ligaments at this point.

such activities must be kept in perspective with the overall mechanical principles. This is not to say that a robust attitude to high performance should not prevail, only that the rider should be aware of the responsibility he takes for the safety of the horse. Fitness and training of both horse and rider are paramount in balancing the risk of injury against the rewards.

It is often argued that the horse would not take part in such activities if it did not want to: whilst this is largely true, every rider knows that successful training is a combination of carrot and stick tactics, which manipulate the horse's behaviour towards his, or her, own ends. Whilst the amount of manipulation required varies between different horses, it is still manipulation. Although the horse may enjoy the activities, it cannot reflect on the potential dangers and make decisions for itself about the risk element. There is thus a moral responsibility to put the safety and well-being of the horse as a first priority.

Muscles and tendons

Muscles are made up of bundles of fibres laid against each other. The strength of muscles is directly a result of the stresses that have been put against them. They develop in response to exercise; regular exercise will develop muscle, and if there is no exercise they will atrophy and become weak.

The development of muscle power is a very important element in the strength of a horse. Muscles, under the influence of stimulation from the nervous system, have the power to contract; and it is this which controls the tendons and in turn the bones, giving the limbs and the whole body motive power. The real power of the horse emanates from the physical contractions of muscles. Having said this, we must not underestimate the importance of the nervous system in this process. Anything which adversely affects the nervous system can cause associated muscles either to lose effectiveness or to become useless.

While muscle tissue is very strong, tearing of some of the fibres is not uncommon through over-zealous exercising. Very occasionally they may also be ruptured by the same process. More common is the rupture of the delicate blood vessels which occur around muscle tissue. Recovery from such injuries will obviously depend on the nature and severity of the problem. Slight problems are sometimes best left to their own devices to heal, but more severe injuries will require assistance and advice from a veterinary surgeon. Problems associated with the legs of horses should be treated with great care, because of the stresses and strains put on them during work. Effective treatment is best carried out by those with a full appreciation of the principles involved.

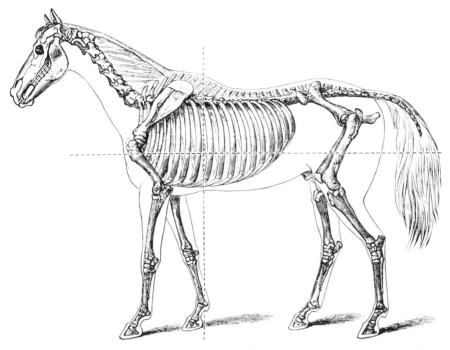

The centre of gravity of the riderless horse is at or near the spot where the lines cross. It is changed by the weight and position of the rider to a point which is higher and further back. If this shift is not adjusted for, by both the horse and the rider, they may be thrown off balance and part company.

The tendons are fibrous, inelastic pieces of connective tissue, attached at one end to the extremities of muscle and at the other to the relevant bone structure. Ligaments are of similar structure and form as tendons, but some have a degree of elasticity. Ligaments differ from tendons in that they connect bone to bone, holding structures together. They are not connected to muscles. Tendons are not in themselves the power of the contraction, but simply the means by which the contraction is transferred to the limb. Whilst they are extremely strong, and their anchorages to both muscle and bone is very firm indeed, they can lose their condition if under-exercised. Like muscle, they benefit from regular exercise to keep them supple and strong. They must be kept in the best possible condition if they are to be fit to bear the strain of hard work. The tendons of the limbs, especially the lower limbs, are particularly important, and their condition should be taken into consideration for different types of work. It should also be taken into consideration that some horses are more suited to certain types of work than others.

Strain on tendons and ligaments obviously increases along with the type of exercise performed. Eventing and racing are probably at the top of the list. Many horses which are just not cut out for the types of stresses involved in, say, eventing will be perfectly good for, and may well excel in, other disciplines: 'horses for courses'.

The respiratory system

The act of breathing air begins at birth and continues involuntarily throughout life. It is so intimately connected with the continuance of life that we often refer to the 'first' and the 'last' breath. However, the simple but vital process of breathing often goes unnoticed, and its importance is often overlooked.

The respiratory process is concerned with the absorption of oxygen into the body and the expulsion of carbon dioxide. Every tissue in the body develops carbon dioxide as a waste product which must be eliminated. The muscles are particularly associated with production of carbon dioxide.

The blood both carries oxygen to the muscles and other organs, and conveys carbon dioxide away from them. This is a simple gaseous exchange and it is reversed when the blood reaches the lungs, which expel carbon dioxide in exhalation, and on inhalation the blood is re-oxygenated and re-circulated in a continuing cycle. The blood is circulated throughout life by means of the heart. The higher the oxygen requirement of the body, for instance during exercise, the higher the heart beat and breathing level become.

The athletic muscular vigour of the horse is necessarily associated with large volumes of air and a highly developed respiratory system. During exercise it must be capable of effecting the necessary exchange of gases. In fact, the horse demonstrates an interesting adaptation to the effects of sustained strenuous exercise. His muscles, under these circumstances, are not able to obtain from the lungs all the oxygen they require. As a result of a change in biochemistry or metabolism an 'intermediate' process occurs, and the immediate oxygen demand from the lungs is thereby reduced.

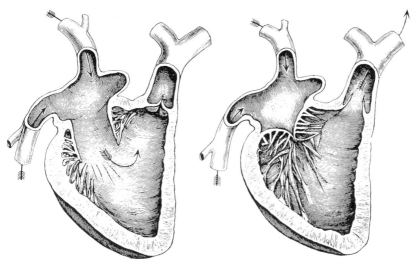

The heart is composed of elastic muscular tissue which is stimulated by the nervous system to circulate blood around the body. The illustration shows the direction of blood flow, and the action of the valves which control the direction of the blood by opening and closing.

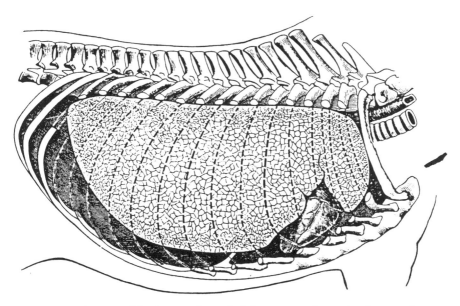

The size of the lungs reflects their importance in moving large volumes of air during respiration. They fill the chest cavity above the heart, the right lung being slightly larger than the left. Adequate blood supply to the lungs is of great importance, not only for absorption of oxygen and elimination of carbon dioxide, but also for proper nourishment of the lungs themselves.

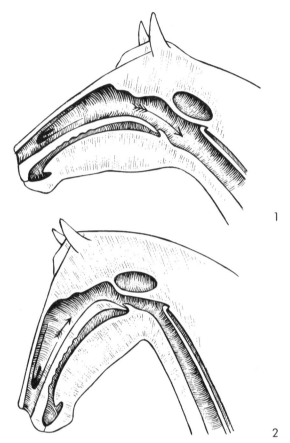

Air intake and different head positions. 1 shows natural head position of a horse at exercise, with clear air-flow to the lungs. 2 shows how a head position fixed by the rider can restrict the air-flow in the pharyngeal area. This can have an adverse effect on anatomical structures as well as limiting air volume reaching the lungs.

However, when the exercise is over, the lungs are able to 'repay the debt' and supply the necessary oxygen to complete the metabolic process.

The chest of the horse is largely occupied by the lungs, which are constructed to offer a large surface for contact with the air. They are often described as being of a spongy texture, and while this is a fair description of their appearance, it can be misleading. The blood continues to be contained within the system – it is only the gases which are allowed to permeate the extremely fine tissue of the lungs themselves. Sound lungs are important to the delicate

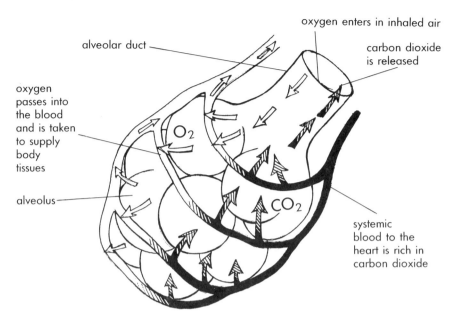

oxygen enters in inhaled air

carbon dioxide is released

alveolar duct

oxygen passes into the blood and is taken to supply body tissues

O₂

alveolus

CO₂

systemic blood to the heart is rich in carbon dioxide

Blood flow and gas exchange in the lung. Oxygen passes into the blood and is taken away to supply body tissues. Carbon dioxide is brought back to the lungs via the circulation and returned into the air by exhalation. During exercise, there is an increase in circulating blood volume from a reserve supply in the spleen.

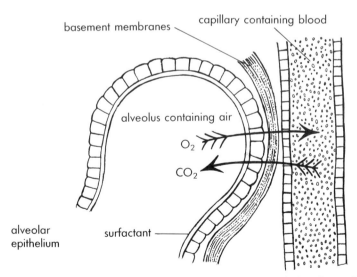

basement membranes

capillary containing blood

alveolus containing air

O₂

CO₂

alveolar epithelium

surfactant

Detail of gas exchange between air and blood. This shows the delicate layers which permit the exchange of gases. Oxygen (O_2) passes from the alveolus to the capillary blood, and carbon dioxide (CO_2) is released back into the air.

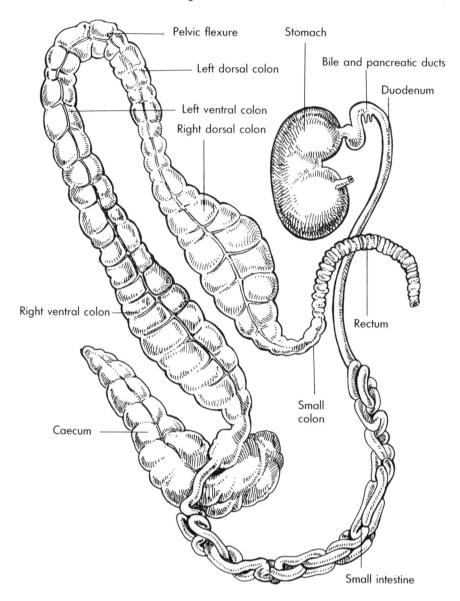

Pelvic flexure

Stomach

Left dorsal colon

Bile and pancreatic ducts

Duodenum

Left ventral colon

Right dorsal colon

Right ventral colon

Rectum

Caecum

Small colon

Small intestine

The major organ for the digestion of roughage (the horse's natural diet) is the large intestine. This contains a large population of bacteria or gut flora which break the food down for absorption by the body. The goodness the horse derives from the food depends intimately upon the composition of the flora. Changes in the population can have a negative effect on digestion and also on health.

and vital nature of this process, which will be impaired by any physical obstruction on the linings of the lungs. Any foreign materials entering the lungs and respiratory tract will irritate their surface, resulting in the production of a watery discharge, which is a natural reaction to facilitate the disposal of the material. This reaction will be produced by the inhalation of dust particles which may or may not be contaminated with moulds, bacteria, or other disease organisms. If these are not discharged efficiently by the natural defence processes, complications may set in which will compromise the efficiency of the gaseous exchange even further. Air quality is vital to the maintenance of efficient lung function.

The digestive system

The horse's lips with their attendant whiskers are a wonderfully prehensile and sensitive structure, useful for locating and assessing the herbage he wishes to eat. The mobility and power of the lips is extraordinary, and the ability of the horse to 'see' with his lips should not be underestimated, such is the tactile nature of this part of the horse's anatomy. It is for this reason that the barbaric practice of de-nerving the nose and lips in the case of head-shakers is totally inhumane and should be disallowed forthwith.

The teeth are open rooted, in other words they are constantly growing from the roots in order to compensate for the wear and tear by the coarse and siliceous material of the horse's natural diet. The front teeth play a less important part, but together with the lips and tongue are used to get hold of food and bring it into the mouth. The crowns of the cheek teeth meet, like millstones, and the action of the jaws provides the grinding action. The tongue plays an important part in determining the amount of chewing required, and also keeps the food between the teeth. The teeth occupy a large proportion of the face, the shape of the head being greatly determined by the need for a structure upon which to mount the teeth, which illustrates their importance for survival.

Proper function of the teeth is vital both to health and to life, not only for safe and effective digestion to take place, but also for mouth comfort and for balanced locomotion. Bad teeth can lead to difficulties with the bit, uneven tension on the neck, unequal loading on the forelegs, and even gross mouth pain. They can also give rise to imperfect digestion, with resultant sub-optimal health or sometimes colic. Regular dental attention is often necessary in the modern horse, since his unnatural diet and life-style lead to abnormal wear patterns. Poor tooth form and function can arise from receiving insufficient fibrous food, too much compound food or cereals; and from eating lush, fertilised grass. If a tooth root becomes infected, this can lead to infected sinus with malodorous nasal discharge. Great skill, understanding and hard work are needed to ensure that the teeth are functioning properly. Annual or in some cases six-monthly attention is needed on a preventive basis.

Stomach

The stomach is not unlike the simple stomach of the human and dog, apart from one or two points. Some degree of fermentation can occur in the stomach, and, because of its shape, the horse cannot vomit.

The inlet to the stomach and the outlet from the stomach to the intestines are close together. Any abnormal distension of the stomach can lead to a blockage of both orifices, effectively sealing the stomach and leading to dangerous colic. In the stomach some soluble ingredients of the diet may be absorbed by the bloodstream, and some basic digestion of simple protein can also take place.

Intestines

The small intestine is able to absorb basic protein and some carbohydrate material. The bulk of the diet passes on to the large hind gut, or colon, and is digested by a fascinating bacterial population within the gut called the bowel flora. The horse provides the bacteria with a home, and the bacteria convert the food into nutrients for the horse – a perfect symbiotic relationship. What nutrients the horse receives as a result of this process depends to a large extent upon the products of the bacterial fermentation. The exact nature of the bacterial population is in turn dependent upon the food being given. We are able to alter the make-up of the bowel flora by changes in the diet, and the goodness derived by the horse from the food depends intimately upon the composition of this flora. Sudden changes in this population can lead to acute poisoning or allergy, associated with colic and sometimes laminitis.

Longer-term effects of an incorrect or unsuitable flora, perhaps associated with unsuitable dietary ingredients or bad dentition, are poor stamina, unthriftiness, an unbalanced immune system leading to susceptibility to infections or allergy, and behavioural problems.

Exercise

Muscles, tendons, ligaments, and the respiratory system may, by gradual and patient increasing of the pressure put on them, be brought to a condition which will properly support hard work. Without such progressive training they would be totally incapable of withstanding the same pressures. The development of the ability to withstand hard work may be regarded as cumulative. Provided that the horse is kept in good condition, it will be capable of gradually increasing its capacity for work as time goes by, until its powers begin to fade due to age. The limiting factor will mainly be the conformation of the animal, assuming saddling, shoeing, and other factors are optimal.

Exercise is central to proper development of the muscles, tendons, ligaments, and respiratory system. Because of the amount of work which we require of horses it is essential to get the muscles firm and the tendons and ligaments as strong as possible, and to develop a vigorous respiratory system. Like food, exercise is regulated according to the amount of work we wish to give the horse.

To develop the horse to its maximum fitness potential, the provision of regular exercise is essential. A horse's legs will suffer less if he is in regular work, simply because they become accustomed to what is required of them. The whole body will become attuned to the rigours of work, developing strength and vigour. It is true to say that horses fit in all these respects probably suffer less from accidents which may arise from over-excitability and over-exuberance.

The power of the lungs is directly connected to the horse's ability to perform hard work. Like the other organs, the effectiveness of the lungs will be improved according to the amount of exercise they receive. Unless the lungs are accustomed to the demands of hard work, they will not be able to perform the function efficiently when required.

Lung function, in this respect, may be regarded as something

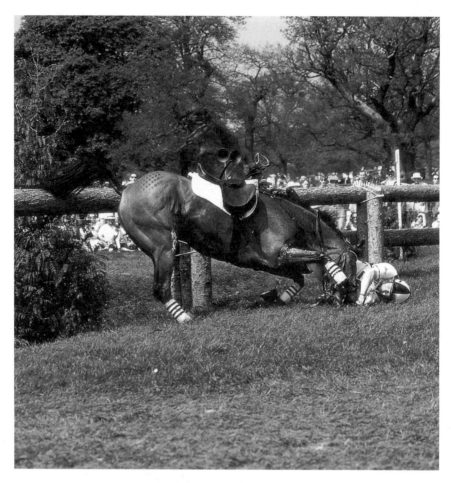

Even with good balance the rider is likely to be unseated if the horse makes an unexpected movement, particularly whilst jumping.

which will follow the demands of the body for oxygen. A horse in good physical condition can be exercised hard in order to get him 'into wind'. Conversely, a horse which is physically unfit can never be galloped into condition.

An illustration of the value of regular work comes from the stage-coach horses of years ago. Many of these animals could not, by any standards, be considered to be of the best conformation. However, they would regularly pull a heavy load at a ten-mile-an-hour trot, for eight or ten miles, without turning a hair. This they would do quite well for many years without any problems.

If exercising the fit horse is suddenly stopped it will quickly run to fat. This is simply because his physiology is now developed to required more fuel. He will continue to consume the fuel, but none will be burned off in work, and the body will store it in the form of fat. Frequently this will be accompanied by other problems involving health.

Getting a horse into fitness depends on many factors. Age, feeding, condition, conformation, and state of the legs must all be taken into consideration, together with an exercise programme which will develop the full potential of the horse without over-working or over-straining him. Whether a horse can reach optimum fitness most often depends on the owner's time available for proper training and exercise.

The relationship between exercise and diet often causes confusion, particularly with regard to modern compound feeds. The rule is to feed according to the level of work the horse is being asked to do. All modern textbooks state this, but it must be seen within the context of total fitness.

'Overheating' is often regarded as a problem, and it is seen as a direct result of feeding. There is no doubt that some foods cause the horse to be more energetic than others — oats have been linked to excessive energy, among other foodstuffs. It may also, however, be a result of the use of inappropriate raw materials in compounded feedstuffs, such as sugars.

In some circumstances it is a good thing to have an extra reserve of energy; in others, not only may it not be required, but it may cause problems. They begin when this extra energy cannot be channelled into a useful activity, often resulting in fractious behaviour caused by frustration. Everything which has the potential for reducing such problems should be considered. Food, work level, training, rider ability, and fitness must all be brought into the equation. The art of good feeding is to take in every factor and remember that all horses are individuals; what may apply to one horse may not apply to another. As with other areas of management, the holistic approach here is to become familiar with the principles involved, by study of both the problem itself and associated subjects. Holistic principles can only be properly applied by taking an overview of the situation.

The training and exercising of race-horses, and other horses which are worked at an extremely hard pace for a comparatively short period, is a specialist subject. These horses must be trained to give of their absolute best at specific times. As with other horses, their fitness depends on the gradual building up of stamina over a period, but it also involves training which must bring the horse to an absolute pitch on a given day.

One of the best ways of monitoring a horse's fitness is by checking the heart beat, which can be done manually at one of various pulse points. The main ones are at the lower jaw, in the hollow of the heel, inside the foreleg at knee level, and behind the elbow. The pulse indicates the force and regularity with which the blood is being circulated round the body. As a general rule, each pulsation corresponds with a contraction of the heart muscle, which is the circulatory pump for the blood.

The volume of blood passing through the arteries is greatly increased during exercise. This is a result of the extra requirement for oxygen. The pulse beat of a healthy horse at rest is about forty beats per minute, although this can vary. The slightest excitement will cause it to alter so the horse should be calm and relaxed if an accurate record is to be made of the pulse at rest. The fore and middle finger should be used across the pulse point, rather than along it. If the fingers are placed in any other way a false picture may be given. The pulse should be regular and strong. By comparing the rate of the pulse after different exercise routines it is possible to determine the relative fitness of the horse. The horse may be said to be fitter if the same exercise routine produces a lower pulse than when previously performed. The rate at which the pulse returns to normal after exercise is also a good indicator of fitness; generally the sooner it slows the better. Regular checks on the pulse will enable the owner to become familiar with the effect of certain exercise routines on the horse, and to monitor the progress of the fitness work-out.

Grooming

Regular grooming is essential to maintain health and condition of the coat and skin of the horse in work. Horses which are turned out and not worked, although they may enjoy the sensation of grooming occasionally, do not require the same amount of attention in this respect because they do not sweat as much as horses in work.

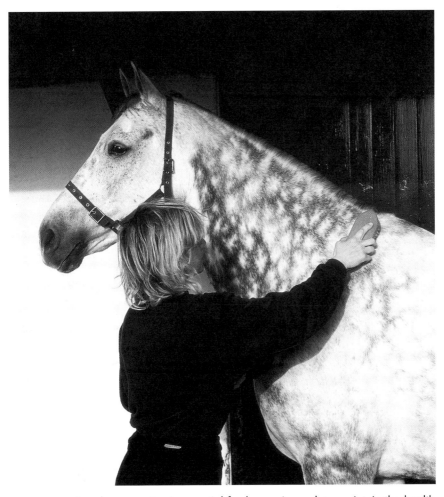

Regular grooming is essential for horses in work to maintain the health of the skin and coat by removing skin debris and dried sweat. It also improves the appearance of the coat.

The amount of work a horse is performing will naturally be reflected in the amount of sweat produced. Horses in hard work sweat profusely. After work, great care must be taken to avoid chills, which can be caused by the effect of evaporation of the sweat reducing the temperature of the skin. Horses with finer and shorter coats may have most of the sweat removed by some drying and cleaning immediately after exercise. Insulating porous clothing may also be used to reduce the chilling effects of evaporation while the coat dries off.

When the coat and skin have dried off, the sweat, together with skin debris, which is a natural sloughing off of dead cells, will have matted into the coat, making it dull and unattractive. Apart from the look of the coat, if the dried sweat and other material is not regularly removed, the function of the pores of the skin will be diminished. As well as making the horse look and feel miserable, it can cause skin problems and actual disease. The other benefits to be had from good grooming is that it discourages the presence of skin parasites.

Initial grooming must be sufficient to reach the skin surface, so as to loosen the debris, which can take quite a hold. This is best done with a stiff bristle brush, and with some vigour, in the same direction as the lie of the coat. Care must be taken not to irritate the skin, particularly in some breeds. Brushing cleans the shafts of the hairs, and the skin surface is invigorated by the massaging action of the bristles. When the process of cleaning the coat and skin by brushing is completed, the surface of the coat may be made more pleasing to the eye by giving it a final polish with a wisp or softer brush.

The use of running water to remove excess mud from the legs is a common practice, and the horse may be shampooed occasionally. To avoid chills, care must taken not to allow the coat to air-dry too quickly when the air temperature is low. This can be avoided either by physically drying the coat, or by the application of insulating clothing, or by a combination of the two.

Insecticidal shampoos are useful, particularly during the summer when flies and other insects may be a problem. The best ones to use are good quality herbal shampoos. It is important to get all the soap out of the coat when rinsing, since if any is left in it may irritate the skin and leave a dull coat. It is a mistake to shampoo too often as coat and skin will become stripped of the essential natural oils, making them dry and unhealthy.

8

Common diseases
and ailments

'Treat the patient as well as the disease.'

Dr Edward Bach (1880–1936)

Most diseases of the horse are man-made, being caused by a variety of interrelated factors. Many can be avoided by following the philosophy of holism. The purpose of the next section is to describe the nature of some common ailments and diseases in order that the reader may appreciate what happens when things go wrong.

Those wishing to follow the principles of holism will probably want to consult a veterinary surgeon practising holistic medicine.* Appropriate holistic medicines and therapies will be prescribed, together with advice for managing the disease and reducing the potential for further occurrence. The type of treatment will depend on the overall medical situation and also on the practitioner.

The relationship between diet and disease will always be considered, and advice will be given as appropriate, as diet is central to good health and the maintenance of the body's innate powers of self-healing.

Some diseases are more directly connected to diet than others, and there is a complex relationship between the two. Treatment should only be sought from a veterinary surgeon, first to ensure the best chance of a cure, and secondly to comply with the law.

There are many predisposing causes of certain problems, for instance the relationship between conformation and some conditions of the limbs and spine. When the musculo-skeletal framework is put under the strains and stresses of work, any mechanical

* The BAHNM will be able to advise on your nearest one.

157

problems which arise will probably be associated with the weakest part of the system. Peculiarities of conformation may lead to weakness in certain activities, and will increase with the intensity of work. The owner should be aware of this and every effort should be made to avoid situations which may store up problems for the future.

Some common diseases and ailments are cited below together with relevant holistic medicine and nutrition. This is a brief overview based on the authors' experience and success in these areas. Some or all of the therapies mentioned may be employed – there is no 'textbook approach' to any problem and treatment will vary greatly in each case. By and large holistic therapy seeks to stimulate healing and maintain health by creating a favourable internal and external environment. Thus although relevant therapies are mentioned, it would not be appropriate to give detailed treatment of each disease. Unlike allopathic medicine which treats one disease with one medicine, holistic medicines and therapies take into account the whole picture. The problem is seen as an accumulation of factors unique to the patient. This means that two horses suffering from the same disease may be treated in different ways.

If proper holistic veterinary methods are not readily available it is vital that other veterinary attention is sought, to ensure that suffering is not caused by neglect of painful or distressing symptoms. An enthusiasm for holistic methods must not be allowed to contribute to poor animal welfare.

Movement

Arthritis

The term arthritis is given to inflammation of a joint. Those commonly affected are the knee, hock, stifle and fetlock. Spavin and ringbone are other manifestations of arthritis. Usually, unless it is the result of a direct trauma, more than one joint is affected. Stiffness after exertion is a common symptom, which may not appear to be a particular problem at first. As the condition progresses, the stiffness becomes worse and swellings begin to appear around the affected joint.

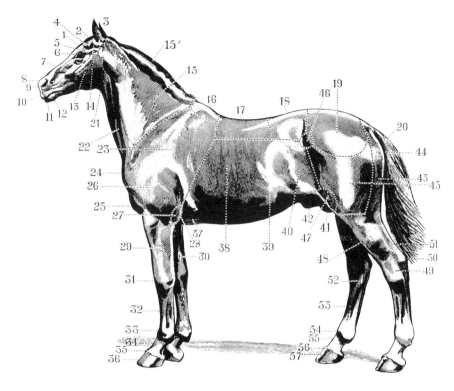

1. Forehead.
2. Forelock.
3. Ear.
4. Supra-orbit.
5. Eyebrow.
6. Eye.
7. Nose.
8. Nasal peak.
9. Nostril.
10. Upper lip.
11. Lower lip.
12. Chin.
13. Cheek.
14. Temple.
15. Neck.
15'. Crest.
16. Withers.
17. Back.
18. Loins.
19. Croup.
20. Tail.

21. Throat
22. Jugular groove.
23. Shoulder.
24. Shoulder point.
25. Breast.
26. Upper arm.
27. Elbow.
28. Point of elbow.
29. Forearm.
30. Chestnut.
31. Knee.
32. Cannon.
33. Fetlock joint.
34. Pastern.
35. Coronet.
36. Foot.
37. Brisket.
38. Chest.
39. Abdomen.
40. Flank.

41. Testicles.
42. Sheath.
43. Buttock.
44. Point of buttock.
45. Thigh.
46. Haunch.
47. Stifle.
48. Leg or gaskin.
49. Hock.
50. Point of hock.
51. Achilles tendon or hamstring.
52. Chestnut.
53. Cannon.
54. Fetlock joint.
55. Pastern.
56. Coronet.
57. Foot.

Points of the horse

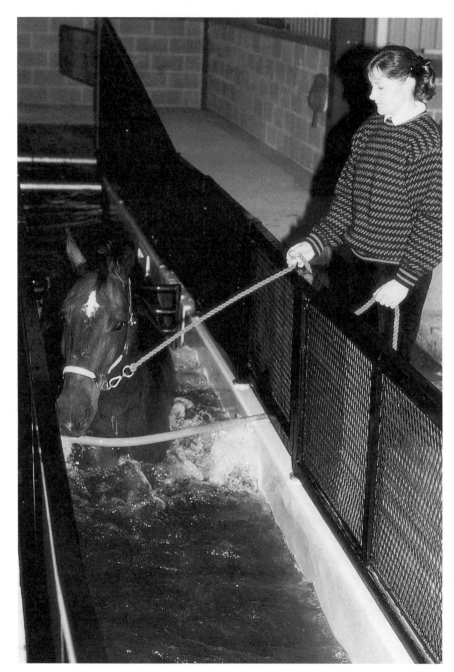

Swimming is a valuable therapy when exercise is recommended as part of a rehabilitation routine, particularly after injuries to the musculo-skeletal system. Also horses appear thoroughly to enjoy swimming for its own sake.

As with many joint problems it may be associated with concussion and hard work or with wrong nutrition. The physical characteristics of the bones of the joint eventually begin to deteriorate, making movement restricted and difficult. Pain and heat in the joint along with lameness will now be apparent. There are predisposing causes of the condition which should be taken into consideration by the practitioner.

Treatment consists of sympathetic management practices which take into account the physical problems being suffered by the horse, together with management of pain. Holistic nutrition and the healing stimulus afforded by acupuncture, homoeopathy and herbs, or a combination of these, can provide effective treatment.

Azotoria

Other names for variations of this condition are 'Monday morning disease', 'tying up', or 'set fast'. Cases may also be known as paralytic myoglobinuria or exertional rhabdomyolysis. The horse develops swelling and pain in the muscles of the loins and hind quarters, and sweats profusely. In severe cases the horse will stiffen up to such an extent that it will be unable to move.

The condition is associated with working horses that are being kept on full rations and stabled. It is also seen in endurance and event horses. Treatment involves the management of pain and other primary considerations together with a gentle return to exercise when appropriate. Holistic therapy in general has achieved success; provision of holistic nutrition is important in prevention.

Back problems

Horses that are not ridden do not get many back problems. The musculo-skeletal system of the horse, like any other creature, is evolved to cope well with the strains that normal activity places upon it. Extra pressure put on the system will cause problems, which will become apparent in that part of the system which is weakest.

The pressure put on the musculo-skeletal system of the horse by the weight of the rider is borne by the whole framework of the body. The combination of the weight and balance of the rider, the work that is being performed, and the physical fitness of the horse has a bearing on the potential for physical problems. Correct saddling is an absolute requirement for comfort and safety and will do much to prevent back pain. While selective breeding can go some way to change the conformation of the horse, and so reduce the potential for problems, the basic mechanical limitations of the body must be observed. The legs are particularly prone to ailments, and so is the back.

The back bears the brunt of the physical weight of the rider, and while it is an immensely strong, rigid structure, it must be protected from undue strain at all costs. Although there are some proportional differences, a good analogy of how a horse feels under a rider is to carry a child aboard for some distance on all fours. If the passenger is relatively still and balanced it is not very hard work, although it may be tiring; however, if the passenger has other ideas, like trying to knock off his fellow riders with a cushion, it becomes a different matter.

Apart from the extra weight, one of the biggest problems is maintaining balance under an unwieldy load. When this happens, the effort involved imposes considerable opposing forces on the spinal column. It might be argued that the human frame was not designed to do this, but neither was the horse's. Of course the attendant risks involved in these activities are multiplied during more energetic exercises and are probably at their highest during jumping.

Apart from the considerations of fitness and rider skill, the other obvious potential for problems is saddle fitting. Currently there is much debate on this issue, but there is one over-riding factor which governs the design and fit of saddles, and that is to minimise the effect of the weight of the rider on the horse's back. Design of the saddle is central to this issue, and the skill of the saddle maker is paramount. Difficulties in this area are extremely common and great care is needed in selecting advice.

Bitting and care of the mouth should also be mentioned here as having obvious potential for causing an unbalanced carriage, which may contribute to back strain amongst other things.

The teeth of the horse should be regularly inspected and rasped if necessary to keep them in good repair. This is particularly important for the older horse. As we have seen, in nature the teeth are kept to the correct length by the constant action of grinding siliceous materials in the diet. Modern feeding stuffs do not provide the correct degree of abrasion so the teeth may become overgrown and uncomfortable.

The common problem is uneven wear of the cheek teeth, or molars, which develop hook-like ridges on the outside edges. If these are not removed it makes the act of chewing difficult and they may eventually cause ulceration. Quidding, when the food is dropped from the side of the mouth during eating, can be a sign that the teeth need attention. Abnormal jaw movements can be detected by observation of chewing or by manual testing.

The wolf teeth, which are the small teeth that grow hard against the premolars, may be removed if they interfere with the bit. Not all horses grow them, and even if they do, they may not cause any difficulties.

The mouth of the horse is a very sensitive part of the anatomy, and by contact with it, along with other aids, the rider is able to maintain control. The bit should lie perfectly on the part of the jaw where there are no teeth, known as the bars, without pinching; if it is properly fitted it cannot be gripped by the horse, or make contact with the teeth.

Many problems which arise, possibly associated with handling difficulties, may be caused by back pain, but may not be recognised as such. The horse may be reluctant to perform some activities, such as jumping, which he knows will hurt him, and this is often misconstrued as bad behaviour.

Back problems are not well recognised in general but are crucial to a horse's health and well-being. Chiropractic help is often very valuable, but one should choose a properly qualified practitioner to work under a veterinary surgeon. Acupuncture may also be of immense benefit. Special exercises can be devised for back health, and once a problem is solved an exercise programme may be instituted; surgery can thereby be prevented.

Capped hock and elbow

Capped hocks and elbows are the result of mechanical damage to the joint. They are unsightly swellings of the synovial fluid, which is the lubricating fluid of the joint. The swelling may be painful to the touch, and normally reduces of its own accord, the synovial fluid being re-absorbed by the body.

The damage may be caused by contact with the stable floor

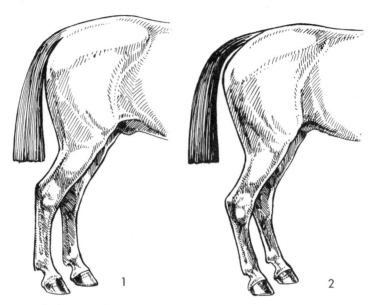

Curby or 'sickle' hocks can predispose a horse to the condition known as curb. In 2 the cannon bone, instead of occupying a vertical position as in 1, inclines forward so that the leg is brought under the body.

caused by lack of bedding and, in the case of capped elbow, by the hind leg kicking at flies during hot weather. Direct trauma can also cause the condition. If it is troublesome seek veterinary advice, as natural medicines can usually help.

Curb

Curb is an enlargement of the plantar ligament which runs down the back of the hock joint. Horses which have a predisposition to this condition are said to have curby hocks. This means that the horse naturally stands with his legs inclined slightly under his body, or stands 'under himself behind'; this causes extra pressure on the hock, particularly the plantar ligament, when the horse is being ridden.

Degenerative joint disease (DJD)

Degenerative joint disease is a generic term for a variety of conditions involving arthritis in the joints. The condition develops for a number of reasons and it is closely related to over-straining the joints during hard work, probably as a long-term result of incorrect gait caused by poor saddling or riding. Nutrition can also play a part.

Over-working the young, rapidly growing horse, and thus putting abnormal loads and pressures on immature joints, is thought to be a contributory cause. This is particularly associated with the racing industry, where financial considerations are paramount in bringing the horses on quickly. Once such predispositions are established, the condition will progress to a greater or lesser degree. Holistic nutrition and medicine are often successful in the management of the problem.

Filled legs

Filled legs is when there is a slight swelling of the lower legs. Both fore and hind may be affected. The swelling is caused by fluid which accumulates under the skin for a variety of reasons. It is usually seen when the horse is first stabled. The swelling has a soft doughy consistency, which is usually quick to disperse when the horse is exercised. There is often no pain or heat associated with the condition and it does not interfere with action, except perhaps for a slight stiffening.

Some horses are more prone to the condition than others and it is thought to be connected to general fitness and nutrition. The cause of the problem is usually multi-factorial and many issues will need to be considered in order to reduce its occurrence. Thus this is a condition which is perfectly suited to the application of holistic principles.

Laminitis

Laminitis is an inflammatory condition of the laminae in the hoof. It used to be known as 'fever in the feet' or 'founder'. The condition is extremely painful, caused by increased pressure of the laminae around the rigid hoof wall, and the horse becomes very lame. The typical stance associated with laminitis is the result of the horse trying to take the weight off the affected feet.

Often the condition is worse in the front feet, so the horse will try to support as much of the weight as possible on the rear. In severe cases the pedal bone is separated from the hoof wall and

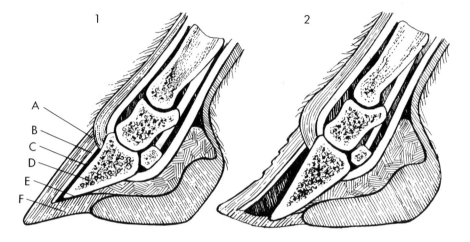

A. Hoof wall.   B. Insensitive laminae.   C. Sensitive laminae.
D. Coffin bone.   E. Sensitive sole.   F. Insensitive sole.

1 shows a cross-section of a normal hoof. Note the position of the coffin bone attached to the laminae and the hoof wall. Laminitis is a condition arising from damage to the laminae which can cause the coffin bone and the hoof wall to separate, as in 2. In severe cases the coffin bone may push right through the horny sole.

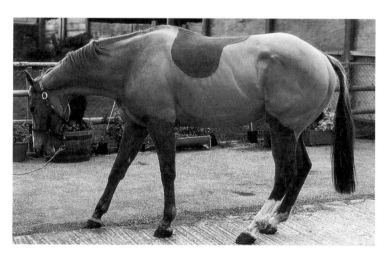

Although laminitis is commonly associated with ponies, it does occur in other types of horses. Here the horse is seen in a typical stance, trying to avoid putting pressure on the affected laminae by leaning backwards. This painful and distressing condition responds well to holistic medicine and nutrition.

rotated from its normal position by the pressure of the deep flexor tendon and the weight of the horse. This causes pressure on the normally concave sole, and in some circumstances the sole can actually be penetrated by the pedal bone. Chronic cases of laminitis will cause the hoof surface to become ridged and deformed, and even if the condition is improved, these outward signs will remain until the hoof grows out.

There are thought to be many causes of laminitis, and it is frequently strongly associated with diet. Holistic therapies are often successful in bringing about a cure when allopathic drug medicine has failed, and may help to prevent further attacks.

Navicular

Navicular disease is a degeneration of the navicular bone in the foot. Simply speaking, the bone acts as a pulley, across which the deep flexor tendon runs. The disease is more common in some breeds than others, being comparatively rare in Arab and pony breeds. There are thought to be several factors which contribute to the condition. Among them are the conformation of the foot associated with concussion, irregular blood supply to the area, incorrect gait due to spinal misalignment, incorrect saddling or riding, and degenerative changes in the bone itself. Skilled farriery is essential in the management of the condition. Egg bar shoes with rolled toes may sometimes be fitted. Holistic medicine and nutrition together with other aspects of management can be very successful in this distressing and difficult condition.

Pedal ostitis

Pedal ostitis is a term that describes an inflammation of the pedal bone. As with all conditions of the foot expert farriery is essential, and appropriate holistic therapy, management and nutrition are usually effective.

Rheumatism

Rheumatism is a general term which is used to describe stiffness and pain in the muscles, joints, tendons or nerves, caused by physiological changes within them. It is associated with predisposing

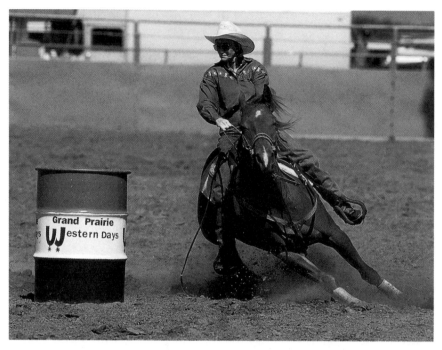

Intense activity such as this puts a high level of sideways stress on leg joints. Proper training and correct diet, among other factors, help to avoid problems such as ligament strain and rheumatism.

circumstances such as injury, old age, and nutritional imbalances. Certain conditions such as damp and cold will often bring on or aggravate the problem. Treatment may consist of reducing the potential for the problem through sympathetic management practices and nutrition, together with natural therapy which will help to resolve the condition.

Ringbone

Ringbone is a bony enlargement of the front, and sometimes the back, of the pastern. It can affect the large pastern bone or the small, and is called high or low ringbone accordingly. It is often seen in heavier breeds and thoroughbreds. Conformation such as upright or long pasterns will predispose the horse to the problem. Any fracture of the pastern bones will also cause the condition, as the bony growth will appear as part of the repair process. The degree of lameness will be dependent on the position of the

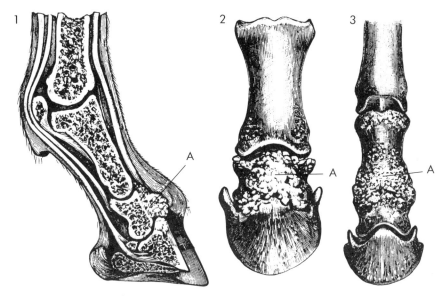

Causes of ringbone are concussion, sprains and mechanical damage. 1 and 2 show low ringbone, 3 shows high ringbone. The abnormal growth of bone is indicated in each case.

ringbone, high ringbone giving less pain than low ringbone. It is caused by concussion, sprains and mechanical damage to the pastern joint. Treatment using herbs and homoeopathy together with sympathetic management and nutrition will serve to prevent further mechanical aggravation of the condition, and may even bring about a clinical cure.

Sand cracks

These are cracks in the hoof wall which either begin at the top of the hoof and extend downwards, or at the bottom and extend upwards. They vary in severity: many horses which develop sand cracks never go lame, others have to be turned away and receive medical attention. The position of the cracks is probably related to the amount of strain that the particular horn fibres are subjected to, and there are positions that are especially likely to be affected, such as the inner quarters of the front feet. The strength of the horn fibres may be affected by nutrition and this should be taken into consideration.

Treatment is usually confined to the prevention of infection, perhaps aided by some surgical and mechanical means to keep the horn from further separation.

Sesamoiditis

The sesamoid bones lie behind the fetlock. When the ligaments holding them are over-strained sesamoiditis develops. The severity of the condition depends upon the degree of strain – in some cases the ligaments are torn, taking a long time to heal. Fracture of one or both of the sesamoid bones themselves sometimes occurs, and is obviously more serious. Fractures of these bones, as with any other, is associated with mechanical stress. General fitness and preparation for the job in hand is the key to reducing the inevitable risks of injury.

Treatment revolves around judicious exercise, laser therapy, holistic nutrition and natural medicines. Serious fractures may require immobilisation to prevent further damage during the healing process.

Stringhalt

Stringhalt is a condition that is thought to be associated with the nervous system. It usually affects the hind limbs. The foot is brought up towards the body in a jerky movement and is held there for a moment, before being forced hard down to the floor again. The muscle spasms responsible for the condition can be brought on by certain movements, such as turning sharply; but they can also occur during slow movement.

The frequency of the condition varies greatly, both in individual cases and between horses. It generally becomes more pronounced as the horse advances in years, or during excitement. Holistic medicine and nutrition and chiropractic manipulation of the spine have been known to help.

Spavin

Bone spavin is arthritis of the hock joint (*see* Arthritis). It involves the lower bones of the joint, and like all arthritic conditions may have many predisposing factors. Conformation is thought to be

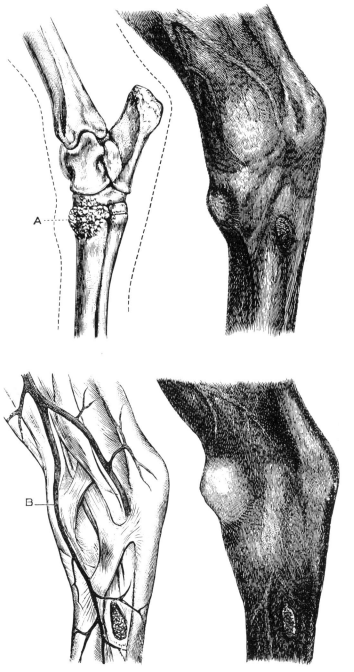

A shows the abnormal bony growth associated with bone spavin. B shows the soft swelling which appears in bog spavin. Both conditions may have similar predisposing factors.

associated with the condition, and strain on the hock joint, particularly during fast exercise, must be suspected.

All joints in the horse's legs are susceptible to strain and damage of some kind. The risk is reduced by fitness training and sympathetic riding practice. Poor saddling will result in abnormal action of the hind legs and predisposal to the condition.

Bog spavin produces a soft, chronic and fluctuating enlargement of the joint capsule of the hock. It appears on the inner and upper part of the joint. The condition is particularly associated with strain, and it is aetiologically similar to bone spavin.

Holistic nutrition and proper saddling, together with the healing stimulus of natural medicines, are usually effective in regaining proper function of the joint and preventing fusion of the small bones.

Splints

A splint is a hard bony swelling which appears under the skin, normally on the forelegs, but they can occur on the hind. They are associated with the splint bone, hence the name. As with many bony problems associated with the legs, concussion can play a part in their development; conformation and balance together with uneven weight distribution is also important.

When splints first develop they may feel hot, and may be painful to pressure, but eventually they settle down to be a cool, smooth, hard lump. The size can vary from something like a pea up to a hen's egg. Treatment depends upon the severity of the problem, and some will resolve and almost disappear without treatment at all. After seven years of age splints are a very rare occurrence.

Tendon strain

Sprains to tendons and ligaments are the result of overtaxing their natural capabilities. Injuries of this sort most commonly occur in competition horses, where damage is often caused to the flexor tendons of the front limbs. Obviously fitness plays an important part in preventing problems, but strains are a risk in any speed event. This risk is heightened in cases of spinal or pelvic misalignment, and if saddling is not correct.

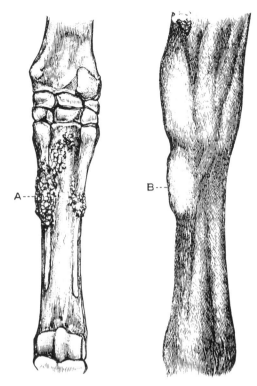

A shows the abnormal bony growth involving the splint bone, B shows the splint covered by skin. The size and position of splints can vary. In severe cases they can cause acute and lasting lameness.

The practice of firing, which is the application of smouldering metal firing irons to the site of injury, was commonly used during the first half of the twentieth century for strains. Its use has fallen out of favour over the years, and it is now obsolete. The theory was that the heat produced a 'counter-irritation' which was supposed to reduce the effect of the injury by diverting the trauma to the new wound tissue. The other benefit was thought to be that the scar tissue so formed would be stronger than the original and act like a permanent bandage.

The practice was thought by some to be beneficial, and by others barbaric. Recent research at Bristol University confirmed that it did not help, and there was no therapeutic basis for its use. The practice is no longer recommended by the Royal College of Veterinary Surgeons. Tendon injuries respond well to laser therapy, proper exercise, and appropriate homoeopathic medication.

Thoroughpins and windgalls

These are soft swellings of the joint capsule. They appear just above and behind the hock and fetlock joints respectively. There are several theories about their exact cause, but they are associated with work in most cases. They tend to decrease in size during work and reappear when the horse has been rested. Apart from being unsightly, they are not regarded as a particular problem by most people. Thoroughpins take their name from the way in which the swelling can be pushed from one side of the leg to the other. Windgalls may arise as a result of poor nutrition, or from immune disturbance, such as adverse reaction to viruses or vaccination. Holistic therapy and nutrition will often help the condition satisfactorily.

Respiratory

Allergies

Allergies are caused by a hypersensitivity to certain agents with which the body comes into contact. Susceptibility to allergies has an association with diet. Dust and pollen allergies are common, particularly in the summer, when crops are flowering; also in the winter when there is an increase in contact with stable dust.

Symptoms include coughing and running eyes and nose, and allergies are also associated with problems such as head shaking and COPD. Treatment includes attention to diet, reduction of exposure to the allergen and natural medicines as indicated by the veterinarian.

Bacterial infections

Some problems caused by bacterial infections of the respiratory tract are pneumonia, bronchitis, sinusitis, and strangles. Bacteria of many kinds exist in the soil and around most stables and indeed houses. Horses and humans come into contact with them every day, and they are part of the natural biological cycles of nature.

In normal circumstances they do no harm whatever to healthy horses, and their presence is not even noticed. Problems begin when the bacteria are able to multiply at a rate which becomes

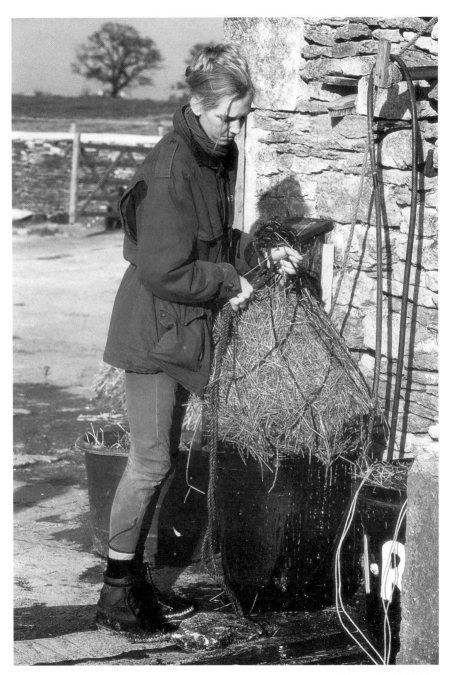

Dust and spores in hay can cause respiratory problems if inhaled by the horse. To keep this to a minimum, hay can be soaked in water for about half a day, then drained and fed before it dries out. The disadvantage of soaking is that it may remove soluble nutrients.

damaging to the body. Routine cleanliness of stables and utensils, plus proper ventilation and reduction of dust, will usually keep bacteria at a level which will be no problem to healthy horses.

Conditions which will allow the bacteria to enter and flourish in the body are typified in a horse with a viral infection, whose natural defences are below par. If the infection is in the respiratory tract, airborne bacteria will be breathed in by the horse, so exposing the damaged tissues to infection. Here they may multiply in an environment that is comfortable to their biological make-up.

An holistic veterinary practitioner will reinforce the body's own defences to such invasions, while directly stimulating its fight against the invading organisms themselves. Good nursing during illness and extra attention to cleanliness and ventilation will go a long way towards preventing bacterial infections of the respiratory tract.

Equine herpes virus

It can take up to three months or so to recover from this type of virus, even if the horse is fit. The symptoms are similar to equine influenza: a runny nose and high temperature are seen, and sometimes the glands of the head and neck become slightly enlarged.

Any discharge from the nose must be regarded seriously, but a secondary infection is revealed by the presence of a muco-purulent discharge, which is thick, discoloured and malodorous. Certain strains of the virus can cause abortion. The same principles of disease management apply as in equine influenza, and similar preventative measures apply.

Equine influenza

Equine influenza is an acute respiratory disease caused by a virus. The incubation period, which is the time lapse between the horse coming into contact with the virus and the onset of symptoms, is short. The virus gains entry into the respiratory tract through the nose and settles in the lining of the trachea and bronchioles. Like all foreign organisms invading the body it settles in that part of the body in which it is most comfortable.

Symptoms of the disease include elevated temperature, coughing, and a nasal discharge. The infection itself clears up in a week or so, with symptoms being worst in the middle of that period. The virus damages the delicate lining of the respiratory tract, but this will usually repair itself within a month or so. Although the virus itself can cause damage to other organs, one of the problems with this type of infection is not so much the virus itself, but the damage it does in terms of laying the way open for secondary infections.

Horses which are susceptible to secondary infections are those which are below par, the young, and the old horse; if a bacterial infection is set up and cannot be controlled, secondary pneumonia may be brought on which in a very few cases can be fatal. The spread of viral infections can be controlled by isolation of the infected horse. Holistic medicines may be prescribed to help clear the mucus, and reduce the risk of secondary infections. Any problems involving the respiratory tract call for adequate ventilation.

Vaccination is often used in an effort to prevent the disease, but can bring on its own problems in sensitive individuals. It should be noted that vaccination is required for many competitions. Homoeopathic and herbal preventative methods can be very effective and safe if carried out under properly qualified veterinary supervision. Proper nutrition is very important to the immune system.

Rhinovirus, adenovirus

In common with equine influenza and equine herpes virus, these two viruses are associated with a runny nose and elevated temperature. Treatment consists of minimising the potential for secondary infections, and ensuring the horse has clean air.

Respiratory viruses, by their nature, produce similar basic physiological problems, therefore their treatment is similar in nature. The different types are characterised by their incidence at certain times or in certain circumstances.

Small airway disease

This is also known as 'broken wind', 'heaves' or COPD. Airborne moulds in stable dust are thought to be the cause. These conditions are often associated with sensitisation, from reaction to viral diseases, or possibly vaccination. As with other diseases of the respiratory tract, good clean air is essential, and management of the disease involves helping the body's own defences by holistic nutrition and medicines.

Intestinal

Colic

Colic is an abdominal pain, and there are several types and causes. They vary in severity from a slight upset, which goes of its own accord, to a life-threatening condition requiring emergency surgery for its relief. The pain is from a distension of the gut caused by a build-up of gas, overheating or a blockage. There are many reasons for colic, but one fairly common one is a change in the intestinal flora, which could possibly be caused on occasion by some of the ingredients of modern compounded feeding stuffs.

Spasmodic colic is, as the name implies, associated with irregular bouts of pain during the attack. These are generally mild in nature, and although distressing for the horse and owner they can be regarded as a slight stomach ache, which will go in time.

During the spasms, the horse will seem tense, and perhaps look round at his flanks occasionally. He will often roll, which will not do harm provided he is not in a position to damage himself. The horse will sweat and the pulse will be raised. The condition will normally last for a few hours or so.

Treatment will include antispasmodic herbs or homoeopathic medication. Acupuncture is also very beneficial. Modern drugs will be required if access to proper holistic medicine is not available.

Tympanic colic is directly related to diet and produces acute continuous pain. High pulse, sweating and a tender abdomen is apparent. Excessive fermentation in the hind gut is the problem, which may be associated with some compound feeding stuffs, certain straight feeds and rich spring grass. The fermentation of these products produces large volumes of gas which cannot escape quickly enough, so producing a tense abdomen and intense pain. Treatment is as above. Some action can be taken to reduce the amount of fermentation in the gut, which allows the natural processes to get back into balance again, using oils and small quantities of turpentine (dangerous in unqualified hands).

Obstructive colic is potentially very serious and it is an emergency condition. As the name suggests it is an obstruction of the intestines; this is often at the pelvic flexure where the intestine narrows near the pelvis. Common causes of obstructive colic are bed eating, consumption of under-soaked sugar beet, or a sudden dramatic change of diet. The obstruction may be an impaction in some cases, or even a torsion, and there is frequently a need for emergency surgery to remove or release the blockage.

Intestinal parasites

Intestinal parasites or worms can be a continual worry for the horse owner. Any parasite which lives inside the body has the potential to damage health. There are many types of worms which use the horse as part of their life cycle; usually the worms enter through the horse's mouth, attach themselves to a part of the intestinal tract in which they are comfortable and remain there, or burrow to other parts of the body until the next stage of development, which usually means being discharged from the body with the faeces. During their period of residence within the horse worms can cause serious problems. Some species cause more physical damage than others.

Common types of worms, each with their own specific modes of action, are bots (fly larvae), pin worms, strongyles, and tapeworms.

An holistic approach involves appropriate pasture and stable management, together with appropriate herbal medicines which can effectively reduce the overall worm burden. Pathological worm burdens are the direct result of intensive pasture grazing and incorrect nutrition. Fencing is the start of the problem, restricting the horse's grazing area. As this is a necessary function of modern life, conventional chemical wormers may prove necessary, even if they do have the potential for harm to sensitive individuals.

Skin

Allergies

Skin allergies cause a reaction typified by physical changes in the skin surface, accompanied by soreness, itching and tenderness. In severe cases secondary infections can be set up.

Sweet itch is one of the most common manifestations of skin allergies. It is mostly seen in pony and cob breeds. The allergy is associated with a midge which bites the horse, which is particularly prevalent during the summer months, June and July being the worst.

Commonly affected areas are the shoulders, loins and rear, particularly the base of the tail. The condition is very irritating to the horse and the affected part may be raw and inflamed, caused by constant rubbing on convenient objects such as trees in an attempt to relieve the itching. The areas affected often lose hair as a result of this and the surface of the skin may ooze serum. Long-term cases will re-grow white hairs on the site of the trauma.

Treatment consists of reducing the exposure to the midges, which is not always practical, together with dietary considerations to reduce susceptibility in future. Non-synthetic fly sprays are available which will repel the midge, and garlic and other herbs may be given to make the coat less attractive to them. The affected skin may be treated by the topical application of aromatic essential oils to deter midges, and healing creams or lotions, containing calendula, for instance.

Urticaria is a condition resulting from sudden changes in diet, such as may be associated with new spring grass. Weals are seen on the surface of the skin, particularly on the flanks and neck. The chances of the condition developing can be reduced if holistic diets are fed, and also if the body is given time to adjust to any changes in grazing.

Photosensitivity is a condition which makes the surface of the skin sensitive to sunlight. The skin becomes reddened and in-flamed and eventually the affected areas become dry and slough off. It is frequently accompanied by hair colour loss. Dietary factors are important: plants such as St John's Wort, when eaten by the horse, can cause the problem via dysfunction of the liver.

All cases of allergies or sensitivities can be helped or even prevented by holistic nutrition and avoidance of sensitising influences, such as unsuitable dietary ingredients, viral infections, or vaccinations in sensitive individuals.

Mud fever, rain scald

Both mud fever and rain scald are commonly associated with similar bacteria-like organisms. Rain scald occurs usually in the winter, when warm, damp conditions of the coat enable the organisms to multiply. Raw oozing patches appear on the surface of the skin. Crusty scabs are then produced, together with matting of adjacent hair.

Being associated with the same organism, mud fever thrives in damp muddy areas. A horse in these conditions will be susceptible to the bacteria as the mud it comes into contact with will abrade the surface of the skin. This gives the organism a hold to begin multiplying and cause infection. It affects mostly the skin on the posterior side of the limbs, but may spread up the leg from the fetlock, and may even reach the stifle and abdomen in really extreme cases.

Since the organism thrives in damp conditions, treatment consists of keeping the area dry and free from further infection. The areas may be gently cleaned before treatment to remove debris and matted hair. Topical application of antibiotic herbs, and creams or lotions to promote healing may be required. These are all available as holistic medicines.

There may be some preventive value in providing a waterproof barrier by using petroleum jelly in susceptible areas; this can only be of value before the bacteria are present. The condition can occur in dry conditions and sensitivity to buttercups may be involved.

Parasites

Common parasites such as lice and mites live in the hair and skin of the horse and can cause intense irritation. Like most parasites they are attracted to these areas because they find them comfortable. There is food in the form of skin debris and blood, warmth from the horse's body, and an environment which is protective. The condition is predisposed by inadequate nutrition and by stress.

Treatment consists of herbal parasiticides to inhibit or kill the parasite, and treating the coat and skin with aromatic repellent to prevent further infestation. Heavy infestations may require dramatic action by some of the more modern pharmaceutical insecticides, which while killing the parasites very effectively, may have other undesirable effects on the horse. Appropriate preventive management such as natural insecticidal washes, holistic nutrition and thorough grooming will help to control the problem.

Ringworm

Ringworm is caused by any of a group of several fungi which spread from horse to horse, or through contaminated tack. The condition is seen as groups of scabby areas appearing raised in rings on the skin, hence the name. Obviously general cleanliness is important in controlling the spread. Treatment is by inhibition of the organism by topical application of appropriate medicines, and by stimulation of the horse's immune system by holistic nutrition and therapy.

Sources of further information

1. The Trading Standards Department will take up any complaints by members of the public, and will act in strict confidence. The address and telephone numbers of local offices appear in telephone directories.
2. The BAHNM operates a free telephone helpline (01252 843282) to give impartial advice on all matters relating to Holistic Nutrition and Medicine. British Association of Holistic Nutrition and Medicine, 8 Borough Court Road, Hartley Wintney, Basingstoke, Hampshire RG27 8JA.
3. The Royal College of Veterinary Surgeons, Belgravia House, 62−64 Horseferry Road, London IP2 1AF, tel. 0171 222 2001, will confirm the names and addresses of practising Veterinary Surgeons.
4. The Veterinary Medicines Directorate, Central Veterinary Laboratory, New Haw, Weybridge, Surrey KT15 1BR, will give information on licensed medicinal products.
5. The British Association of Homoeopathic Veterinary Surgeons, Alternative Veterinary Medicine Centre, Chinham House, Stanford in the Vale, Faringdon, Oxon SN7 8NQ, tel. 01367 710324.
6. British Horse Society, British Equestrian Centre, Stoneleigh, Kenilworth, Warks CV8 2LR.
7. British Veterinary Association, 7 Mansfield Street, London W1M 0AT.
8. Ministry of Agriculture, Fisheries and Food, Ergon House, c/o Nobel House, 17 Smith Square, London SW1P 3JR.

183

References

Clare, John, *The autobiography* (quoted in *Rainbows, fleas and flowers*, ed. Geoffrey Grigson, John Baker, 1971).

Colgan, M., PhD, *Your personal vitamin profile*, Blonde & Briggs, 1984.

Jung, C.G., *Man and his symbols*, Aldus Books, 1964.

Karic, E., *Vitamins: a shelter against disease*, Reshafim, Tel-Aviv, 1975.

Ludwig, H. *et al.*, *Report on distillation product industry*, Eastman Kodak Affiliate Publication, Sept. 1962.

Manning, A. and Serpell, J. *Animals and human society*, Routledge, 1994.

Matsuaka, T., Evaluation of monensin toxicity in the horse, *J. Am. Vet. Med. Assoc.* 1976, 169: 1098.

Mervyn, L., BSc, PhD, CChem, FRSC, *Thorsons complete guide to vitamins and minerals*, Thorsons, 1989.

Mindel, E., PharmB, RPh, *The vitamin bible*, Arlington, 1982.

National Research Council, *Nutrient requirements of horses*, National Academy Press, USA, 1989.

Nature Conservancy Council, second report covering the period 1 April 1975–31 March 1976, HMSO, 1976.

Sharon, M., MD, *Complete nutrition*, Prion, 1994.

Stockwell, C. *Nature's pharmacy*, Arrow Books, 1989.

The Farmer's Magazine. A periodical newspaper first printed at the Strand in London on 15 June 1832.

Youatt, W., *The horse*, Baldwin & Craddock, 1831.

Index